HOPE
FOR
HEALING

*90 Moments with God for Physical,
Spiritual, and Emotional Wholeness*

DR. REGGIE ANDERSON
with JENNIFER SCHUCHMANN

TYNDALE
MOMENTUM®

The Tyndale nonfiction imprint

Visit Tyndale online at tyndale.com.

Visit Tyndale Momentum online at tyndalemomentum.com.

TYNDALE, Tyndale's quill logo, *Tyndale Momentum*, and the
Tyndale Momentum logo are registered trademarks of Tyndale
House Ministries. Tyndale Momentum is the nonfiction imprint
of Tyndale House Publishers, Carol Stream, Illinois.

*Hope for Healing: 90 Moments with God for Physical, Spiritual, and
Emotional Wholeness*

Designed by Mark Anthony Lane II

Published in association with the literary agency of Creative Trust,
Inc., 210 Jamestown Park Drive, Suite 200, Brentwood, TN 37027.

The day 35 devotion, "Seeing His Answer," is adapted from
*Appointments with Heaven: The True Story of a Country Doctor's
Healing Encounters with the Hereafter* (ISBN 978-1-4143-8045-2).
Other devotions were previously published in *The One Year Book
of Healing* (ISBN 978-1-4964-0574-6).

ISBN 978-1-4964-5079-1

Printed in the United States of America

27	26	25	24	23	22	21
7	6	5	4	3	2	1

Introduction

I have written these brief daily offerings to help you meditate on God's healing promises. My hope is that the devotions in this book will encourage you to pursue a closer relationship with him. I want you to see the many ways that he intervenes in the lives of the sick and the hurting, and the many ways that he heals, so that you will be inspired to have hope and faith—to know that God can bring healing to your life. I want you to see what I see every day as I care for my patients—namely, that God is alive and he is active in our lives. I want you to know how much he cares for you.

At the beginning of each devotion, I have included a verse or two of Scripture. But I encourage you to have your Bible handy so you can look up the verses in context to gain a more complete understanding.

Following the Scripture verse, each devotion has a story of healing. Sometimes the story is directly related to the verse; others are stories that came to mind after I prayed about the verse. My hope is that the combination of these verses and stories will show you that our sovereign God is still very much in the healing business. I want to assure you that he loves you and desires for you to be whole and healthy—though sometimes we won't experience complete healing until we join him in our forever home. Even when healing doesn't happen as quickly or completely as we may desire, I hope these stories demonstrate that God is always present in your pain and suffering. My patients continue to amaze me with stories of how their faith has grown, even when their prayers weren't answered the way they hoped they would be.

At the end of each devotion, I offer a suggestion (Today's Rx) for something specific that you can do or consider that will make you feel better, grow stronger, or draw closer to our Father. Then I close in prayer.

The personal stories from my own life and medical practice are all true. But to protect the privacy of my patients, I have changed their names, circumstances, and other identifying information. After three decades of practicing medicine, I have seen many similar cases dozens of times, so some of the stories are composites of details from different cases. Conversations have been reconstructed based on my best recollections.

The medical information provided in this book is specific to the patients I saw in my office or in the emergency room. The treatments prescribed are not intended to diagnose, cure, or treat anyone else's medical or health condition. It is not medical advice and should not replace the advice of your physician. Please consult your doctor to determine what is right for you and your situation.

And while I am adding disclaimers, it would be wise for you to consult with your pastor before following my spiritual advice, as well. After all, I'm not a theologian; I'm just a country doctor.

I hope the stories in this devotional will convince you that the healing hand of God isn't limited to the pages of the Bible. Our Lord continues to heal the sick and hurting today. I have seen his extraordinary work in my own life and in the lives of my patients. My prayer is that you will see God work in your own life, as well.

Dr. Reggie Anderson

THE BEST TIME TO START IS NOW

My child, pay attention to what I say. Listen
carefully to my words. Don't lose sight of them.
Let them penetrate deep into your heart, for
they bring life to those who find them, and
healing to their whole body.

PROVERBS 4:20-22

Do you remember the last time you visited a doctor
or a counselor? After discussing your ailments, the
practitioner likely gave you a set of instructions to
help you feel better.

When you left the office, you were committed to
implement the recommended plan. But maybe that's
as far as it went. Maybe life got in the way, and before
you knew it, the doctor's advice had been shuffled to
the bottom of your to-do list. A week later, you had
forgotten you even had a plan. The advice that had
once seemed important enough to consult with and
pay a professional for had somehow slipped away.

The all-too-common pattern of wanting answers
to our problems but never implementing them can
also happen with God's Word. We go to him looking
for wisdom and guidance, but even when we receive
his instructions, we file them away for a day when
applying them seems more convenient. But the
right time never seems to come. We all have good
intentions, but we're lacking on the follow-through.

We keep putting off until later what we should do right now. When we procrastinate, it often means we never get around to what is important.

If we really want the life and healing that God promises, we can't let his wise words slip away. If we lose sight of God's wisdom, it's worse than if we had never received it. We need to abide in God's Word, allow it to penetrate our hearts deeply, and put into action the things we've heard God say. Write down what God has said, and place reminders where you won't lose sight of them. That is how they will penetrate deeply into your heart.

TODAY'S RX

Has God asked you to forgive someone? Call that person now. Has God asked you to give something? Give it now. Has God asked you to show love to someone? Love that person now.

Lord, thank you for giving me wisdom and counsel through your Word. Help me to draw from it daily, impressing your instructions upon my heart and applying your words to the problems I face.

DAYBREAK'S FRESH START

The faithful love of the LORD never ends! His
mercies never cease. Great is his faithfulness;
his mercies begin afresh each morning.

LAMENTATIONS 3:22-23

Growing up on a farm, I learned that the early
morning was the best time to get things done, before
all the distractions of the day began to clamor for
attention. As a doctor, I have continued that habit.
For many years, I got up at 5:00 a.m. and drove
twenty miles toward the eastern horizon, watching
the sunrise and reflecting on how God's mercies are
new every morning.

At the big-city hospital, I was usually one of
the first doctors on the floor making rounds. This
allowed me to get reports from the night shift nurses
and greet the oncoming day shift. And because it was
early in the morning, I also had the opportunity to
speak with my patients as they woke up to hear about
their dreams and how they had slept.

Medically speaking, the early hours of the morning
are the most common time of day for a heart attack,
stroke, or pulmonary embolism. This is due in part
to low cortisol levels during the night and a sudden
rise in blood pressure when the patient first awakens.

The greatest stories of God's mercy often came
during the night, and I was first on the scene to get
the full picture. Even though morning is a critical

time of day, it is also a time of joy, with the opening of new opportunities. The sunrise sheds light on the darkness of the night. Daybreak brings renewed hope of another day of healing.

TODAY'S RX

Watch tomorrow's sunrise; it's the sweet spot of the day.

God, thank you for each new day, for every breath that fills my lungs, and for every sunrise that reminds me of the hope I have in you.

THE POWER OF PRAYER

Are any of you sick? You should call for the elders
of the church to come and pray over you, anointing
you with oil in the name of the Lord.

JAMES 5:14

We've all had times when we've been sick. Whether
we had a minor cold or something more serious, we
learned how miserable we can feel when we're under
the weather. With proper care and rest, we typically
recover fairly quickly, and even those with chronic
or debilitating illnesses would say they have good
days along with the bad. But there's one thing that is
always true: When we're sick, we want to feel better.

In today's key verse, James describes the
importance of praying for healing when we're sick.
Many Christian churches have a formal time for
these kinds of prayers. Other churches may be less
structured and more spontaneous as needs arise,
but they are nonetheless committed to this practice.
Having people pray for us when we're sick helps us
to feel better. It's a sign that people love us when they
will intercede with the Great Physician for our well-
being. But prayers don't only help us to *feel* better;
they can also help us *get* better.

In medical literature, there is scientific evidence
that patients who have people surrounding them
with love and prayer generally fare better than those
who don't. Patients who have been prayed for recover

faster, report less pain, require less medication, and have fewer complications.

As a doctor, I've been at the bedside of many patients when elders from their church have come to pray for their healing. And I've personally seen many patients with severe illnesses recover and return home to their families and continue living fruitful lives.

I've also been at the bedside of many patients when prayers for healing were not answered as hoped, and we had to trust God for his higher purposes. But even when those illnesses ended in death, the process of praying brought emotional healing and comfort to those who were present. It's as if we were able to catch a glimpse of the patient's soul completely healed on the other side of heaven's veil.

TODAY'S RX

Whatever kind of healing you need—spiritual, emotional, or physical—ask others to join you in prayer today for your healing.

God, thank you for the comfort of bringing my requests to you and knowing that you hear me and love me. Where I am weary, please bring healing and strength, and help me to fully trust in you.

STRONG AND COURAGEOUS FOR THE FIGHT

Be strong and courageous, all you who
put your hope in the LORD!

PSALM 31:24

"He just doesn't seem as strong as before. He says it hurts to run and that he doesn't feel well. He used to want to play outside all the time, but now he wants to stay in."

Tommy's mom was concerned. Tommy was only five, and he'd started losing weight and having night sweats.

"It's the middle of winter, and he's burning up every night. Last year he had strep. The year before that, both ears were clogged, and you sent him to get tubes in his ears. Do you think it could be one of those problems again?"

Tommy looked pale, and he was thinner than I remembered. When we weighed him, he'd lost five pounds—a significant amount in a child that young.

"Hmm. Let's look and see." I got my light out. "His throat looks good. Ears look good—the tubes have fallen out, and his tympanic membranes are normal." I felt his neck and could tell that his lymph nodes were enlarged. They were also enlarged in his armpits. "Let's get some lab work done and see if that will tell us anything."

When the blood work came back, it gave us a

definitive answer—but one we had all hoped and prayed against. Tommy had acute lymphoblastic leukemia (ALL), cancer of the blood and bone marrow. I joined hands with Tommy and his mother, and we prayed, "Lord, this diagnosis is not what we'd hoped for, but now that we know the answer, help us to fight this battle. Give us courage and strength, Lord, for our hope is in you."

The next year was a difficult battle for both Tommy and his mother. The treatments seemed to last a lifetime, but he made it through. Tommy is now in remission with about an 85 percent chance of a cure.

In the midst of adversity, the Lord answered our prayers and gave both Tommy and his mom the strength and courage they needed during his fight.

TODAY'S RX

We all have areas in our lives where we must fight. Place your hope in the Lord, and ask him to provide you with the strength and courage you need to make it through.

Lord, sometimes the road ahead is daunting, and I'm overcome by the challenges I face. Help me to trust in you for courage and strength during these times of trial.

PERSISTENCE IS NOT A PROBLEM

Everyone who asks, receives. Everyone who
seeks, finds. And to everyone who knocks,
the door will be opened.

MATTHEW 7:8

"I've got a problem, and I was wondering if you could help me," Drew said. "It seems kind of silly, but my wife—"

"Your problem is your wife?" I asked.

"No," Drew said, laughing. "My wife thinks I may have a problem, but I'm not so sure. I'm here because she made me come, and I'm hoping you'll tell me it's not a big deal."

"Sure. What's up?"

"I have a spot on my back, near my right shoulder. My wife pointed it out a few months ago. I thought it had always been there, but she said it hadn't. Now she thinks it's growing, but I think it's pretty much the same size—of course, I can't see it that well because it's on my back. It's not painful or anything, but she won't let it rest until I hear from you that it's nothing to worry about."

"All right, let me take a look," I said.

I noticed the spot immediately. It had signs of melanoma—irregular borders, with different shades of brown and black.

"Well, Drew, I think your wife is right to worry

about it. I know you're a farmer, and farmers can get a lot of sun even when they're not trying. I think it would be wise for you to have a biopsy done."

I sent him to a dermatology department that specialized in melanoma. The report confirmed my initial diagnosis. Drew and his wife both came in to get the results. "We're going to storm the gates of heaven with our prayers," she said after hearing the news. She also wanted a list of the best oncological surgeons. "I'm going to call around and get as many answers as I can, and we'll just keep praying until God makes each step clear."

"Drew, it looks like your wife is looking out for you. Not only was she persistent about getting you in here, but I have a feeling she'll be even more persistent in her prayers for you."

TODAY'S RX

Is there something irregular in your life? Don't wait until it causes you pain; pray about it now. When it comes to prayer, persistence is not a problem.

God, help me to pray frequently and fervently, lifting my worries to you, knowing that you will hear me and answer me. Thank you for listening and keeping me under your watchful care.

MEDICINE CHANGES, GOD DOES NOT

Whatever is good and perfect is a gift coming
down to us from God our Father, who created
all the lights in the heavens. He never changes
or casts a shifting shadow.
JAMES 1:17

I have practiced medicine for more than thirty years.
Occasionally, I've reflected on the exponential growth
of and changes that have occurred in medicine during
that time.

Recently, while cleaning out an old filing cabinet,
I found some notes I'd taken while in medical school.
For the better part of an hour, I sat on the floor and
read through them. I laughed out loud about some
of the things I'd written down. At the time, the
gold standard advice and treatment we were told to
give our patients seemed rock solid. But with new
discoveries, many of those solid rocks had crumbled
under the weight of new evidence.

For example, my notes contained information on
an antibiotic that was the recommended first line
of treatment for a certain infection. We now know
that this treatment is totally ineffective. It used to
be thought that peptic ulcer disease was caused
by stress. We now know that it is often caused by
the Helicobacter pylori bacteria, and it's treatable
with antibiotics. Back then, MRIs were still on the

drawing board; we had never seen one. Now we use them daily to diagnose problems that weren't detectable even a few years ago.

As our knowledge of medicine grows, it seems that the ground we once stood on continues to shift. The one and only constant in healing is God himself.

The same prayers of hope and healing prayed for patients thirty years ago, fifty years ago, one hundred years ago, even one thousand years ago, are still heard at the bedside here and now. God never changes. Even in our evidence-based world of medicine, he is, has been, and always will be the gold standard in healing.

TODAY'S RX

God heals, and God never changes; but with the advancement of human discovery, he may change the tools he uses to heal us.

God, in this ever-changing world, thank you for remaining constant from the beginning of time. You are and always have been a loving, gracious Father who hears and answers prayers.

PASSING ON
THE BLESSING

After Jesus left the synagogue with James and
John, they went to Simon and Andrew's home.
Now Simon's mother-in-law was sick in bed with
a high fever. They told Jesus about her right away.
So he went to her bedside, took her by the hand,
and helped her sit up. Then the fever left her,
and she prepared a meal for them.

MARK 1:29-31

Simon's mother-in-law was lying in bed with a
high fever, and Simon was very concerned about
her. I'm sure the other disciples were, too, but let's
face it, they were probably a little disappointed.
They had planned to spend the night at Simon's.
They were expecting an evening meal and a place to
sleep. But with Simon's mother-in-law in bed, their
choices became limited; they couldn't have a pizza
delivered or order Chinese takeout. In addition, they
had to be worried about catching whatever it was
she had.

When I receive a call from the hospital or nursing
home staff, the first thing I do is ask about the
patient's temperature. God created our bodies to heal
themselves when something goes wrong; and in its
simplest form, a fever is often a sign that the patient
is fighting an infection.

But in the ancient world, before aspirin and

antibiotics, a fever could signal a life-threatening illness. In fact, the fever itself could be life-threatening.

That's why it was so important for Jesus to go directly to the bedside of Simon's mother-in-law. There, he took her hand and helped her to sit up. Immediately the fever was gone, and she was able to get up.

Think about how complete this healing was. Most of us, when we've been sick, will still be fatigued and in need of rest, even after the fever is gone. But Simon's mother-in-law felt good enough immediately to get out of bed and begin preparing a meal for everyone.

I believe she did exactly what Jesus wants all of us to do. When he blesses us, whether financially, with good health, or in some other way, he wants us to pass that blessing along to someone else.

TODAY'S RX

For your own good health, pass along a blessing to someone else.

God, you've shown me your great love through the kind acts of others when I've been sick. Please help me to do the same, shining your light and love on those in need.

Day 8

WHY DOES GOD ALLOW TRAGEDY?

The LORD is close to the brokenhearted; he rescues
those whose spirits are crushed.

PSALM 34:18

During the first fourteen years of my life, my faith
in God was innocent. It wasn't built on struggle or
hardship, and it had never been tested. My life was
pretty sheltered, and I was happy. I believed God
was all-powerful and ever present. The role models in
my life all demonstrated grace and kindness, which
further reinforced my belief that God was good.

And then, one horrible day, my close friends
(and distant cousins) Jimmy and Jerry Alday were
senselessly murdered, along with several of their
family members. Jimmy, Jerry, and I had worked
summers together selling watermelons at the Atlanta
State Farmers Market, and those two hardworking,
God-fearing men had a tremendous influence on my
life and faith. And in an instant, they were gone.

For a long time after that, I accused God of
turning his back on his people and not being
powerful enough to take care of them. *Where were
you when the Aldays were murdered?* I silently raged.
Why didn't you protect them?

During the summer following their deaths,
I spent hours at the market sitting alone with my
memories, frightened by the prospect of evil. Heaven,

which had once seemed as close to me as the wind in the trees, now seemed unapproachable. Sin had new depths, depravity had new meaning, and I felt vulnerable to the darkness.

My big brothers and earthly protectors were gone, and I was no longer certain that my heavenly Protector could be trusted. In fact, God seemed useless to me now.

It took years for God to woo me back to himself. Only as the Lord began to soften my heart did I recognize that he had been with me all along. Why hadn't I seen or heard him? Could it be that I had been the one to turn away from God just when I needed him most?

Over the course of my life and practice, I've learned that God does not willingly harm his people; rather, he is a God of infinite compassion. In times of grief, I encourage you to turn *toward* God instead of away from him.

TODAY'S RX
Ask God to help you see and celebrate his glory where it shows up—in the midst of pain as well as in joy.

Father, thank you for being a God of infinite compassion. Help me to keep my eyes focused on eternity and to celebrate your glory in the midst of pain as well as joy.

HEART DISEASE AND DISEASE OF THE HEART

"O LORD," I prayed, "have mercy on me. Heal me,
for I have sinned against you."

PSALM 41:4

Sickness has many causes. Unsanitary conditions, genetics, poor diet, lack of exercise, and lack of proper medical care can all cause disease or worsen the outcome of an illness. When sin entered the world, it not only separated us from God, but it also caused or contributed to many of the conditions that foster disease and illness.

Today, with our knowledge of biology, we put up a good fight against many of these disease contributors, but we often don't consider another cause to our pain that modern medicine can't treat.

When a patient complains of heart pain, sometimes it's not a physical problem—it might be better described as a heartfelt pain. The heart is suffering, but it isn't sick from a disease; it's sick from a lack of repentance or reconciliation. Whether the cause of the pain is a broken relationship with a loved one, private anger aimed at a coworker, or unmet dreams and desires, the illness isn't seated in the body; it's in the soul.

This kind of sickness can create legitimate medical symptoms such as stress, high blood pressure, increased cortisol levels, or chest pain. Though these sins of the spiritual heart can lead to real physical disease, the root of the problem is that the patient's sin is interfering with the person's healthy relationship with God.

If you recognize these soul symptoms in your life, the first step to a healthy relationship with your Creator is to ask for forgiveness. It's a simple step in his treatment plan, but it's a hard one for many people to take. When you ask for forgiveness, you can know that God's forgiveness is complete and his healing starts immediately. His treatment brings peace and hope for the future. That's where the journey to both spiritual and physical health begins.

TODAY'S RX

A doctor can perform a checkup on your body, but you have to perform a spiritual checkup on the condition of your heart and soul.

Lord, forgive me for the anger and resentment I harbor in my heart. Help me release this weight I've been carrying, and wash me clean with your Word.

ORDINARY FAITH HEALING

I have pleaded in prayer for you, Simon,
that your faith should not fail.

LUKE 22:32

When Anthony received a diagnosis of renal cell carcinoma, he called me for advice.

"What do you think about my going to the Mayo Clinic for treatment?" he asked.

"Half the success of any treatment is the patient's belief that it's the right plan. If you want to go to the Mayo Clinic, you should go."

I knew his only real chance for long-term survival was a complete and clean surgical removal of the cancer, and Mayo would do a great job.

A few weeks later, I saw Anthony sitting in his truck with a big grin on his face. "Hey, Dr. Anderson!" he called out. "They got it all. I just wanted you to know."

"That's great to hear," I said.

A year later, Anthony went back for a checkup and found the cancer had returned. The doctors removed three lymph nodes.

"We'll just keep praying for God's will," I said, knowing the news wasn't good.

"But I need to tell you something else," he said. "One night, around two o'clock in the morning, I woke up and started praying real hard, asking God to heal me. Suddenly, a man and a woman stood at the foot of my bed. They said to me, 'How do you know you haven't already been healed?' And then—I know this is going to sound weird, but—"

"Tell me," I said. "I've experienced a few weird things of my own."

"As they left, the wall suddenly opened up right next to them, and for about two minutes, I got a glimpse of heaven."

"What did you see?"

"It was the most beautiful garden with vibrantly colored flowers. I felt as if I could reach out and touch it, but then it was gone."

"Anthony, that sounds a lot like what I experienced in a dream one time."

"No matter what happens to this body, my faith has been strengthened, I know I've been healed, and I don't have any more fear."

"I know what you're talking about. God gave you a glimpse of home."

"But, why me?" Anthony asked. "I'm just an ordinary guy. I don't even know Scripture that well."

"I don't know, but I know that the disciples were just ordinary guys until they met Jesus too."

TODAY'S RX

In his wisdom, God may give you a glimpse of your forever healing.

Thank you for revealing yourself in unexpected ways, Lord. You never fail to astound me by showing me glimpses of your glory. I long to experience more of you.

GET A LITTLE R&R, NOT A TOMBSTONE WITH RIP

Why am I discouraged? Why is my heart so sad?
I will put my hope in God! I will praise him
again—my Savior and my God! Now I am deeply
discouraged, but I will remember you.

PSALM 42:5-6

Three chemical systems in the human brain—serotonin, norepinephrine, and dopamine—help us stay balanced emotionally. God created our bodies to have checks and balances, as well as backup systems to keep us healthy emotionally and physically. However, we were not created for a broken world. We were made to live in paradise. So there are times when our environment seems to overwhelm even our backup systems.

At times it can seem as if the world is spinning out of control. The days rush by, and the more we do, the more we feel we must do. We never seem to get enough rest. I think the rat race is especially bad in the United States, where the American Dream has become more of a nightmare. Depression affects more than one-third of the population to the degree that they will need outside help at some point.

There is no shame in needing help. And there is no shame in stepping aside to take care of yourself. I tell my patients the same thing I tell myself: Make time to recover from the battle. We all need to get some R&R (rest and relaxation), or we'll end up with an RIP sign over our resting place.

God knows we occasionally need a break from the world. That's why he wants us to rest in him. He wants us to sing songs from happy and hopeful hearts. The writer of Psalm 42 asks many of the same questions we ask, but ultimately he knows that his hope is in God. At night when he is discouraged, he sings songs of prayer and praise. This ancient practice is the same thing that will help us live happy, balanced lives even when we have a chemical imbalance.

Commit to getting out of life's rut and seek others to hold you accountable. Restoring your soul might be as easy as sitting quietly and enjoying the simple things in life.

TODAY'S RX

Sadness is commonplace, but you don't have to live there. You are not alone. Help is available. Step outside yourself to find someone who can help.

God, reveal to me moments in my day when I can take time to be quiet and rest in you. Place on my heart a desire to be in your Word, and help me to find my hope and joy in you.

THE SOURCE OF
ALL COMFORT

All praise to God, the Father of our Lord Jesus
Christ. God is our merciful Father and the source
of all comfort. He comforts us in all our troubles
so that we can comfort others. When they are
troubled, we will be able to give them the same
comfort God has given us.

2 CORINTHIANS 1:3-4

When our son, David, was born, he had a double
cleft lip and palate. We grieved for the pain and surgeries we knew he would have to endure. But we
also knew that God had given him to us for a special
reason—even though at the time we didn't know
what it was.

David's first two years of life were full of doctors'
visits, hospitals, IVs, and surgeries. During that time,
Karen and David bonded in a deep and meaningful
way. Not only was Karen his mother, but she was also
his protector, nurse, and voice when he had none.

After the last major surgery for his palate, the
plastic surgeon mentioned that he often met with
young parents who would soon be going through
the same things we'd just finished. He asked Karen
if she would be willing to meet with them and share
her experiences. Being the giving soul that she is, she
emphatically said, "Yes, of course!"

When the plastic surgeon called occasionally with

the details of a new patient, Karen would arrange to meet with the young parents and their baby. Whenever she went on those visits, she took David with her as a living sign of hope for the parents to see that, in a few years, their babies would be healed as well.

Usually during these visits, Karen shared David's story and comforted and reassured the parents. Most visits ended with prayer for the parents and their baby—that God would give them all strength and courage to face the battle ahead.

I marveled at how Karen was able to comfort others, but I also knew the reason why—God had first comforted her. Because of her experience, she knew what others in the same situation needed. She was a willing vessel ready to pass on God's comfort to those who needed it most.

TODAY'S RX

If you need comfort, seek God, the source of all comfort. If you see others who are struggling, share your struggles. Empathy can be a great source of comfort.

Father, you've shown me your faithfulness time and again by comforting me during tough times. Help me to live out your example and be a comfort to my friends and family.

THRIVING LIFE

Fear of the Lord leads to life, bringing security
and protection from harm.
PROVERBS 19:23

My dad taught the agriculture classes at the high
school I attended as a teenager. I took one class
from him in which I learned the names of all the
woodworking tools, and I built a set of bookcases for
our home as a final project.

Two other students worked together to build a
greenhouse, and it was quite impressive. Walking
through the plastic veil was like walking into another
world. On the inside, they had created their own
miniature Garden of Eden.

Inside the security and protection of the
greenhouse, the plants grew perfectly. Because of
the barriers to the outside, there didn't appear to
be any bugs. They could control the temperature,
the amount of food, and the water each plant
received. Disease, if it existed, was limited. Inside the
greenhouse, the plants did more than just survive;
they thrived.

It wasn't surprising to me that all the farmers
in Plantersville wanted one. Those students kept
building until they had filled our tiny town with
more than one hundred greenhouses!

Today's verse says that fear of the Lord leads to
life. In Hebrew, the word for "life," *chay*, means to be

alive, green, and overflowing like a waterfall. When we call upon God, he wraps a protective barrier of safety and security around us, and he gives us just the right amount of love and nourishment to lead us to abundant life. As our love for him grows, we are perfected in much the same way as plants in a greenhouse. Though intruders and disease may enter our world, they can't devour us because God is in control.

TODAY'S RX

If you're trying to survive on your own, turn to the Lord and you will thrive.

Father, put up the necessary barriers in my life to protect me from harm. Allow me to thrive in your presence. I desire to grow and mature as a believer and to be a beautiful creation in you.

THE JOY OF LIFE AND DEATH

This is a sacred day before our Lord.
Don't be dejected and sad, for the joy
of the LORD is your strength!
NEHEMIAH 8:10

When I was young, funerals were sad events. It was hard for me to say good-bye to a loved one. Whether it was my friends who were murdered or beloved grandparents who had died, I missed those who had gone on before me.

As a doctor, I have grieved with parents who lost children much too early. When a child dies, the whole world seems out of order and upside down. Those events are forever seared into the parents' hearts and memories. They lose their ability to think rationally. Their joy in life is lost in a torrential, enveloping storm of grief.

But if we believe in Jesus, we know that what awaits us on the other side of that threshold is the Savior who died to forgive us of all our sins—past, present, and future. He is standing there with outstretched arms awaiting our arrival. On heaven's side of the veil, there is no sickness, sadness, or dejection. That is truly something to look forward to and celebrate.

When I was asked to speak at my father's funeral, what came to mind were all the memories I had of a great man who had lived a good life. Of course, I was going to miss him, but I rejoiced in the fact that he was now in heaven.

It's easy to focus on death. But life isn't about when we will die; it's about how well we will spend the time that God has given us here and now. We may celebrate the fact that we temporarily cheated death by surviving an accident or recovering from a terrible disease, but the only way to experience the pure joy of heaven is to step across the threshold of death.

My father fought the good fight. As I spoke of his life, it brought encouragement and hope to all of us who were there to celebrate him. We want to make the most of our time here on earth, but we also look forward to the joy of one day being reunited with those who have gone before us.

TODAY'S RX

Find joy in life today, and make every moment count.

Father, help me to fight the good fight and live whole-heartedly for you. May my words and actions reflect you and be life-giving to those around me.

TRUST YOUR PROVIDER

For the word of the LORD holds true,
and we can trust everything he does.

PSALM 33:4

I have often seen medical treatments prescribed to patients that should work, but for some reason, they don't. I've also seen treatments that shouldn't work because they had no scientific basis, and yet they work; the patients thrived and got well.

Why does the same treatment plan or medication work for one person and not for another?

What's the difference between treatments that work and those that don't?

I believe it has to do with whether the patient trusts the treatment plan and the doctor who prescribed it.

Nearly every medical study—whether testing a new treatment or a new drug—is tested against a placebo (no medical treatment). Though a placebo doesn't have any medical value, it always results in a positive response for some people. In other words, doing nothing works just as effectively as the medicine or treatment that is being tested. This is called the placebo effect. The reason we see the placebo effect work positively is because patients who don't know they are receiving the placebo believe that whatever they are taking works. In some cases, the response rate to the placebo can be as high as 30 percent.

That's the kind of faith God wants us to place in him and his words. When it seems as if nothing is happening and there is no proof that we are receiving what we think we need, he wants us to trust his Word. If we believe in God's Word, he is faithful to keep the promises he has made to us, and he's proved this over and over again, not only in the Bible but in our lives.

As today's verse says, the word of the Lord holds true. If faith in a placebo works 30 percent of the time, imagine what 100 percent faith in God can do!

TODAY'S RX
Trust God. He still keeps his word.

God, you are faithful, and your Word always proves true. I know I can go to it for the answers I need. Help me to seek your truth above all else and come to you first for counsel.

Day 16

HEALING WORDS

Some people make cutting remarks, but the words
of the wise bring healing.
PROVERBS 12:18

Thirteen-year-old Carly was a good student, excelling
in all her classes. Her mother spent her days as Carly's
full-time academic coach, doing everything she
could to help her daughter gain entry into an elite
university. Though admission to college was still years
away, Carly's mother talked about it so much during
her appointment that I became concerned that she
wasn't taking time to just enjoy being Carly's mom.

During one of Carly's annual exams, when her
mother stepped out of the exam room to take a
phone call, Carly looked at me and said, "Can I talk
to you while my mom is out of the room?"

"Absolutely," I said, sitting down next to her.

As my young patient struggled to put her feelings
into words, I sensed that something was wrong.
After a long silence, Carly blurted, "My mother
thinks everything has to be perfect. If it's not, she
snaps at me."

Once Carly had worked up the courage to speak,
the words came tumbling out.

With tears pooling in her eyes, she described how
her mother's controlling behavior and occasional
outbursts made Carly feel helpless and out of control.
The pressure to live up to her mother's high standards

was immense. I noticed that Carly's nails were bitten to the quick, and she was slightly underweight for her height.

"Tell me about your weight," I said.

"I know, I'm so fat," Carly said. "When I look in the mirror, all I see is a big blob."

I decided that an intervention was necessary. I referred Carly to a pediatric psychiatrist at Vanderbilt Medical Center who specialized in eating disorders.

Over the next few months, God intervened as well.

Both Carly and her mother began the long process of redemptive healing. They attended counseling separately and together and followed their counselor's advice. Carly started eating regular meals and worked to have a balanced lifestyle.

Year after year, I followed their progress as the two women became emotionally healthy. Eventually, they celebrated Carly's admission to an Ivy League school. By her own choice, Carly had surpassed every goal her mother had set for her. She's now in medical school, studying to become a psychiatrist.

TODAY'S RX

Before you speak, remember the wise words of Bambi's friend Thumper: "If you can't say something nice, don't say anything at all."

Lord, let my words build others up today, not bring them down. Help me to reflect the kindness of your Spirit and be a source of encouragement and light to them.

WE WORK BECAUSE OUR HOPE IS IN THE GREAT HEALER

We work hard and continue to struggle, for our
hope is in the living God, who is the Savior of all
people and particularly of all believers.

1 TIMOTHY 4:10

"Code 10, Room 7. Code 10, Room 7."

In the blink of an eye, a sleepy Sunday morning in the emergency room went from calm to controlled chaos as staff members grabbed instruments and equipment and organized under my direction. Though it may have looked like bedlam, it was well orchestrated, with each professional doing his or her part. My role was to be the maestro with the baton, calling in the other players at the exact moment when their skill and expertise were required. Leading the charge to save the man's life, I gave my orders:

"Chest compressions at 100 per minute."

"Breathing pattern ratio of thirty compressions to two ventilations."

"Charge the paddles to 360 joules. Clear . . ."

"Continue compressions."

"Epinephrine IV. Charge the paddles to defibrillate a second time."

When the man's heart was finally shocked back into a normal sinus rhythm, the staff and I breathed a collective sigh of relief and offered silent prayers of thanks. The patient could finally be moved to the ICU.

Before everyone returned to normal duty, I thanked each member of the code team. Without their professionalism, dedication, and experience, the outcome would not have been the same. Furthermore, I knew that each person believed he or she was there to serve a much larger purpose.

I am proud to be a part of a group of Christian health professionals who understand that God is the one who ultimately heals. We're blessed to be his hands and feet—occasionally used to carry out his healing work—and we're blessed that he utilizes our gifts for his glory. Though I may have directed the players, God orchestrated their lifesaving talents and their instruments into a symphony of healing. In playing our respective parts, we all had a role in something bigger than ourselves.

Where in your own sphere of influence is God able to use the gifts he has given you for his purpose and his glory?

TODAY'S RX

If God ever calls you to use CPR, just remember that 100 chest compressions per minute is the same rate and rhythm as the Bee Gees' song "Stayin' Alive."

God, help me to be your hands and feet so that I may reflect your goodness and love to those around me. May I use my gifts well and bring you glory.

Day 18

HOW LONG?

I am on the verge of collapse, facing constant
pain. . . . Do not abandon me, O LORD.
Do not stand at a distance, my God. Come
quickly to help me, O Lord my savior.
PSALM 38:17, 21-22

"How long will it take until I feel better?" It's
something we all want to know when we're not feeling
well. Have you ever asked that question and received
a less-than-satisfactory answer? Maybe your doctor
wasn't forthcoming with a prognosis, or maybe the
specialist, after looking at your test results, was afraid
to tell you that your condition might not improve.

Chances are, if you're in pain, you've already
considered what life might be like if you never feel
any better. What hope is there in a situation that
doesn't promise an end to the pain?

As a doctor, I've treated patients with chronic,
debilitating, and progressive illnesses. For some of
them, there is no cure or answer this side of the veil.
In those cases, I do my best to prescribe medication
to take the edge off the pain and to allow the patient
to live life as fully as possible. Even in the direst of
circumstances, I don't want anyone to give up hope
for healing.

I've often found that even when people's bodies
are wracked with pain and their hope in the health-
care system is declining, their faith in God may be

vibrant and growing. Frequently, at these times, patients find new hope and a renewed appreciation and love for family and friends. They develop a deeper longing for, and trust in, our heavenly Father. The trust they once reserved for their doctors and medical science is now fully placed in God.

If you're suffering right now, I pray that God will lift up your weary soul and give you strength for the day. I pray you will take each day and each breath with the knowledge that he loves you and that he is in control, even when you're struggling. Though healing may not be available for you here and now, hope is still accessible. If you trust in Jesus, one day, in the blink of an eye, you will have a new pain-free body, and the suffering and anguish of this world will be gone.

TODAY'S RX

When your pain has no end, take one breath at a time, and know that your suffering can draw you closer to Jesus.

Jesus, I don't always understand your ways, especially when I'm hurting and my world seems upside down. Reassure my heart of your love in these moments, and fill me with your presence.

Day 19

THE HEALER WHO STILL DRAWS CROWDS

That evening after sunset, many sick and
demon-possessed people were brought to Jesus.
The whole town gathered at the door to watch.
So Jesus healed many people who were sick with
various diseases, and he cast out many demons.
But because the demons knew who he was,
he did not allow them to speak.

MARK 1:32-34

Everywhere Jesus walked, he could always draw a crowd. Amid the masses, there were always those who needed healing and those who sought spiritual understanding. Not much has changed in two thousand years.

A missionary friend of mine from Ecuador called after he received a copy of the *JESUS* movie in Spanish. For some time, he had been praying for an evangelical tool he could use in the villages where his medical caravan went to heal the sick. He was delighted to discover that the movie presented the gospel concisely in a way the villagers could understand. He asked me to come see the impact for myself the next time I could make it to Ecuador.

The weeks leading up to that trip were full of preparations. What I needed to pack depended on where we were going, so I waited for my friend's call.

"We've been invited to go to a remote village at 14,000 feet, so prepare for snow and ice," he said.

"Really?" I asked, confused. "Snow and ice at the equator?"

A few days later, we set up camp and a makeshift clinic in the main mud hut of a mountain village. At night, the whole town came out to watch the *JESUS* film. Most had never seen a movie, and they were amazed by the modern technology. They came out of curiosity, but they left with a fuller understanding of who Jesus is.

There was a great outpouring of the Holy Spirit through this film project. Many were spiritually saved, and some were physically healed. I was astonished and amazed to see ancient scenes of the Bible come alive right before my eyes. Crowds still gather to see Jesus, and he still has the power to render us speechless.

TODAY'S RX

Run to Jesus. He still heals.

Jesus, I have no doubt about your power. You continue to make yourself known in remarkable ways across the world, bringing new life to people of all backgrounds. Thank you for loving your children so well.

Day 20

A HEALTHY AND GLAD HEART

No wonder my heart is glad, and my tongue
shouts his praises! My body rests in hope. For you
will not leave my soul among the dead or allow
your Holy One to rot in the grave.

ACTS 2:26-27

"It's kind of late for a farmer to be sleeping in, isn't it?"

Brett opened his eyes, yawned, and smiled. He was usually up and out before the rooster crowed, but he'd had heart surgery the day before and was still recuperating.

Brett had grown up on a meat and potatoes diet—usually with dessert to polish it off. And like many of my patients whose diets had placed them at an increased risk for premature heart disease, his unhealthy eating habits had caught up with him. At forty-two, he was much too young to have undergone heart surgery.

"Brett, your heart surgeon gave me a call yesterday. That surgery saved your life. He said you needed a four-vessel bypass and that you had a 99 percent blockage in the left coronary artery—that's what we call a *widowmaker*. You're a lucky man to have this much heart disease and not much muscle damage."

"I am thankful," Brett said. "That widowmaker almost caused me to meet my maker! But I know that God has a different plan for my life."

"You're right. He does, but you're going to have to make some different choices about your health—specifically, your diet."

"I know. You've been preaching to me about diet, exercise, and especially watching my portions. Being in the ICU gives a man a lot of time to think. I realize that instead of my friends and family gathering at my bedside right now, they could be gathering at my graveside. Not only am I going to make changes, but I am going to make sure everyone I know realizes they need to make changes too."

Brett was faithful to his word. He made a major overhaul to his life and became an evangelist to his friends and family, not only for God's goodness, but also for good health. Each day, when he gets up before the rooster crows, he thanks God for his second chance.

TODAY'S RX

When faced with a major blockage in your heart or in your soul, look to God for a way to bypass the damage and start a new life.

Lord, you are a God of second chances, allowing people to be reborn into new life with you. Thank you for not giving up on me, and instead showing me the way.

GOD'S ODDS

This hope will not lead to disappointment.
For we know how dearly God loves us,
because he has given us the Holy Spirit
to fill our hearts with his love.

ROMANS 5:5

At forty-three, Mark had every reason to live and yet one reason that might prevent him from doing so.

Mark's daughter was getting married in six months. She had planned her wedding for the following year but moved up the date when Mark was diagnosed with pancreatic cancer.

Fortunately, the cancer had not spread, and the oncology surgeon felt that Mark might have a chance of surviving with something called the Whipple procedure—a major surgical operation involving several organs. If Mark hoped to be at his daughter's wedding, this was his only option. Without it, the odds of surviving this type of cancer for more than a few months were close to zero.

As we talked about possible complications and outcomes, Mark asked me, "Will I be going through the motions just to get to the end of it all and still have cancer? Could I end up dying anyway before the wedding?"

With God, I believe there is always hope for healing, but I never want to give my patients false hope in medicine. So I gave Mark my honest assessment.

"Dr. Paulo is one of the best, and I trust his judgment in this area. I don't think you'll be disappointed with your decision. But this journey isn't going to be easy."

At Mark's six-week postsurgical checkup, he was twenty pounds lighter and beginning to eat without pain. "I wouldn't suggest this as a diet plan," he said, "but if it gets me to the church for my daughter's wedding, I'm glad I went through with it."

A few weeks ago, Mark was back in my office for his annual checkup, and he was unusually talkative. "When I went through my surgery, my family loved me even when I was at my worst. I'm beginning to understand God's love for us because I saw it reflected in my family's love for me during those dark days."

"How long ago was the surgery?" I asked as I flipped through his chart.

"It's been three years, and not only was I able to walk my daughter down the aisle, but last month I received another gift."

Mark handed me a photo.

"My grandson!" he said, grinning.

TODAY'S RX

With God on your side, the outlook is always favorable.

Holy Spirit, fill me with your presence today. Help me to have a positive outlook on all I'm facing, and give me hope for my future.

GOD MAKES THE WEAK STRONG

Hammer your plowshares into swords and your
pruning hooks into spears. Train even your
weaklings to be warriors.

JOEL 3:10

I had been asked to stop by the nursing home to
see an elderly patient who had become despondent.
Catherine had recently had a stroke, but I knew she
could recover from it. The problem was that she
didn't seem to want to.

When I entered the sparsely furnished room,
Catherine looked ashen and pale—a rag doll wrapped
in twisted sheets. She pulled the covers over her head
when she saw me. I glanced at the nurses, and they
nodded. Everything about her demeanor suggested
she'd given up.

"Why are you hiding from us?" I asked. "We're
just trying to help you."

Catherine mumbled something that I couldn't hear.
Her voice was barely audible—more like a whisper.

The reason she didn't feel well had nothing to
do with her stroke. She and Thomas, her husband
of fifty years, had lost all their valuables in a flood a
few years earlier. And recently, Thomas had gotten
ill and died.

"I know you want to join Thomas," I said, tenderly
taking her hand. "But your time hasn't come yet."

The stroke hadn't taken her life, but it had certainly disrupted it. Her speech was distorted, and the right side of her body was now weakened and crumbling before our eyes.

"God has further plans for your future with us. He wants you to pick up your plowshare and hammer it into a sword and fight for this new journey—this plan for your life." I wasn't sure why I said those words, or what they meant to her. But I hoped they would encourage her.

As we continued to talk, she took her fist and pounded the bed. After a few minutes, she pushed herself up and got out of bed. When I left, she was sitting in a chair by the window, where the sunshine could pour into her soul and dry her tears.

Catherine wasn't transformed overnight, but God definitely performed a miracle in her life. I saw it, and so did the nursing staff. Catherine hammered away at her recovery until she was well enough to return home, strengthened and ready for battle.

TODAY'S RX

Never give up, and never give in to the whisper of despair. When you're weak, allow God to make you strong for the fight.

Father, help me to keep my eyes on you when I'm weighed down with grief. I know it is when I am weak that you are strong. Thank you for revealing yourself in new ways to me during this time.

ALL IT TAKES
IS A GLIMPSE

Always be full of joy in the Lord.
I say it again—rejoice!
PHILIPPIANS 4:4

When I was on vacation in Venice, Italy, I sat in the Piazza San Marco and watched the tourists entering and leaving St. Mark's Basilica. The cathedral has opulent gold mosaics throughout, which have earned it the nickname Chiesa d'Oro, or Church of Gold.

The tourists I saw all had such joy on their faces! I'm sure they were delighted to catch a glimpse of the basilica's splendor. As I watched, it made me think, *This is how we should live our entire lives—full of joy, wonder, and worship.*

My mind wandered to thoughts of Jesus' disciples—how they had lived their lives and how most were martyred for their faith. *Did they live lives full of joy?*

Eleven of the twelve apostles died by some form of execution. They must have struggled and suffered much more hardship than we, who live in a world of comfort and convenience, could ever imagine.

Yet throughout their days on earth and even at the untimely moment of their deaths, their hearts were filled with joy. I have to believe that, no matter what happened to them, no matter how bad their days were, their eyes were fixed on their forever home in heaven.

When I find I'm having a difficult day, I try to think about eternity in paradise worshipping the Father, Son, and Holy Spirit. As I reflect on the delight I observed on the faces of the tourists who visited the ornate cathedral at St. Mark's, I imagine the freedom and joy we would have in our lives if we focused on our future in eternity.

I pray that God will give you a heavenly glimpse of our Promised Land to help sustain you on your bad days. With each passing day, we know it won't be long before we join him there.

TODAY'S RX

Resolve to live today in joy, knowing that you are one day closer to the joy of your forever home.

Lord, I give this day to you, promising to approach it with a joyful spirit and glad heart.

A PILL AND A PRAYER ARE BOTH GOOD MEDICINE

A cheerful heart is good medicine, but a broken
spirit saps a person's strength.

PROVERBS 17:22

"No matter what I do, I'm tired all the time," Beth
said. "Even when I try, I can't seem to get up before
noon. What do you think is causing all of this? Last
night, I was looking at my symptoms on the Internet,
and it kept saying that tiredness could be caused by a
problem with my thyroid or that I could be anemic.
Do you think that's the case?"

Beth looked worried. She also looked tired. "We'll
do some blood work to assess those possibilities," I
promised. "But first, start by telling me about your
sleep habits."

"Usually, I go to sleep around midnight or one,
but most nights I can't fall asleep, so I get back up
and try to do something until I get tired."

"What else is going on in your life?"

"I don't know. I feel as if all I do is worry about
what's going to happen next. They're laying people
off at my husband's workplace, and I'm afraid he
could be next. When he's under stress, he doesn't take
good care of himself, so I worry about his health. The
kids haven't been doing very well in school, and my
mom hasn't been feeling well. Also, next month I'll

be working a lot of overtime—and I'm not looking forward to that."

I was starting to get the picture. Though Beth was certainly busy, there was a lot more going on with her emotionally—and her anxiety was keeping her awake at night. Her fatigue was probably not due to a physical cause but rather a worried heart and broken spirit.

As promised, I ordered some tests and lab work, and it all came back perfect, as I had anticipated. After I explained to Beth that there didn't seem to be a physical cause for her exhaustion, we discussed some options for dealing with her anxiety. She decided to try medication and prayer.

Within two months, I could see the positive results of both. I knew she was on the mend when she bounded into my office and started talking about all of the great things the Lord was doing in her life.

TODAY'S RX

When worry and the cares of the world break your spirit, turn to the Lord to find joy, hope, and peace.

From day to day, God, there are always new concerns and worries. Be with me when my heart panics and my thoughts become a jumble. Calm me with the truth of your Word, and help me to remember how you've always been faithful in the past.

PRUNING FOR A FRUITFUL LIFE

If you remain in me and my words remain
in you, you may ask for anything you want,
and it will be granted!

JOHN 15:7

As a small boy, I used to watch my father prune the peach trees in our orchard. Even when I was very young, he taught me how to tell the difference between the branches that produced fruit and those that were diseased, dying, or already dead. The unhealthy branches could safely be pruned because they would never produce fruit. By the time I was a teenager, I could finger a branch in the dead of winter and know whether it had life teeming inside it or if it would only divert resources from the rest of the tree.

The branches that remained after pruning were our hope for a bumper crop, and we did whatever it took to protect them. If a late freeze was expected, we built a fire in the orchard to ward off the cold. During the growing season, my father kept an eye on each tree for signs of what it needed. More water? More fertilizer? A little more pruning? He spent countless hours nurturing the trees and protecting their yet-to-be-borne fruit.

Jesus is the watchful gardener who tends to our spiritual health. He sees what we need even before we recognize it. And he is quick to offer us protection.

But unlike a tree, we can decide whether or not we will live and abide in him. Do we allow him to take care of us, or do we think we know what's best and resist his care? Do we have branches that need pruning—areas of our lives that need to be cut away and discarded?

When we allow the master gardener to tend to us, he never reduces our fruitfulness; he only increases our yield. But when we resist his pruning, we end up hanging on to dead, diseased, or sinful areas of our lives that prevent us from being fruitful.

Jesus invites you to remain in him and allow his truth and wisdom to prune your life and make it more fragrant and fruitful than you can imagine.

TODAY'S RX

In medicine, surgery is much like pruning—we cut away the dead and diseased parts. We need to allow the Great Physician to do the same thing to us spiritually if we want to thrive and bear good fruit.

Jesus, thank you for tending to me so carefully, preserving me through harsh seasons and growing me in others. May my life be fruitful and pleasing to you.

Day 26

THE FIRST STEP IS THE MOST IMPORTANT ONE

Jesus immediately reached out and grabbed him.
"You have so little faith," Jesus said.
"Why did you doubt me?"

MATTHEW 14:31

When I ponder Peter's act of faith in stepping out of the boat to walk on the water toward Jesus, I don't think about his walk or his fall. I think about that first step. What kind of courage did it take for him to hoist himself over the side of the boat and onto the water? I've often tried to imagine what he was thinking as his foot touched the waves. Frankly, I'm impressed that he did it; I would have been cowering in the back of the boat!

Sometimes, the first step is the hardest. Many of my patients come to me with an addiction to alcohol, tobacco, or even food. They want to quit the behaviors that are killing them, but they feel powerless. To overcome any kind of addiction, you can't keep doing what you've always done. You have to take a first step toward the life you want. That first step is often to admit that you have a problem and you're powerless over it. You need to ask for someone's help—maybe a friend, a pastor, or a doctor. God can work through many people to show his love for you.

Do you feel paralyzed by inaction? Are there

places you want to go in your life, but you're not sure how to get started in that direction?

The first step is to take that first step.

Whether you sink or swim, you have to get out of the boat and begin moving toward your destination. Fortunately, we know that Jesus is with us every step of the way. If you look, you will see him coming toward you. If you fall, it is his arms that will reach out to catch you. The faith to take the first step is all you need to propel you in the right direction.

Take that first step toward healthy living, and have the confidence that even if you get a little wet, Jesus will be your life jacket.

TODAY'S RX

If you're afraid to step out, at least talk to God about your fear. He can give you the courage you need to move forward.

Jesus, I want to take that first step toward a healthier lifestyle. Help me to stand firm in my commitment and have faith in my ability to persevere. Be with me every step of the way.

PATIENT EXPECTATION

All glory to God, who is able, through his mighty
power at work within us, to accomplish infinitely
more than we might ask or think. Glory to him
in the church and in Christ Jesus through all
generations forever and ever! Amen.

EPHESIANS 3:20-21

Do you often feel as if you're in the waiting room of
life? Does it seem like you've been waiting forever for
the Great Physician to emerge from the operating
room to give you the news you long to hear?

In those moments when we're waiting for an
answer to prayer, the results of a medical test, or the
end of therapy to see if our strength has returned,
we can change our view from one of passive waiting
to one of patient expectation. When we open our
Bibles, we see God's plan and purpose through his
words, which provide us with the comfort we need
to know that all will soon be well because God can
accomplish infinitely more than we might ask or
imagine.

Too often when we pray for healing, we stop
short of asking for all we want. With our weak logic
and feeble faith, we think that if we ask for just a little
bit of healing, God is more apt to answer than if we
were to ask for complete healing. But today's verses
remind us that God's mighty power at work within
us can do more than we think.

I have seen many medical miracles that can only be explained by God's "mighty power at work." Many of these miracles are documented in this devotional and in my first book, *Appointments with Heaven*. In addition to the healings I've witnessed, I have also seen God's power at the bedsides of those who are about to meet Jesus face-to-face.

Both physical and spiritual healing are part of God's plan. We are often shielded from all the reasons he does what he does, but today's verses remind us that he is all-powerful and that all glory belongs to him—even when we're in the waiting room of life.

TODAY'S RX

The next time you're waiting, rather than pacing and wondering, read God's Word and know that he is able to do everything that is within his will.

Jesus, thank you for this reminder that you are capable of more than I can even imagine. I boldly ask for complete healing and a clean bill of health in your name.

ROLLING THROUGH LIFE

I still dare to hope when I remember this:
The faithful love of the LORD never ends!
LAMENTATIONS 3:21-22

"I hear you need some insurance paperwork filled out. How can I help?"

"Ol' Bessie needs a new battery and wheels," Neil said, patting the side of his electric wheelchair. "I've about worn these out."

I looked at the bent rims and worn treads. "Looks like you've been traveling."

"I get around," he said, smiling.

Neil had been a patient of mine since he was in elementary school. He was a good kid but never one to sit still for long. After he graduated from high school, he'd been a promising college student at a nearby university. But that was before the accident.

It all started with a dare. Neil and his frat brothers were out partying one night, and on the way home, somebody bet him that he couldn't get his old Ford pickup up to 100 miles an hour. He had proved them wrong, but he was going too fast as he approached Creekside Curve. Unable to stop in time, he had slid off the road and hit a tree. Now instead of a pickup truck, he drove Ol' Bessie, with a top speed of about four miles per hour.

Bessie might have been slow, but that didn't stop Neil from going wherever he wanted. In the four years since the accident, he'd gone as many places and met as many people as any other twenty-four-year-old I'd known.

"Describe how the accident has affected your daily life," I said, reading from the form.

"Since the accident, I need help with everything. I can push the joystick, and I can talk, but everything else is in God's hands—or in the hands of the angels he's sent to help me," he said, nodding to the young woman assisting him that morning.

"I could have lost my life on that curve, and when I woke up in the ICU, I knew immediately that it was Jesus who'd saved me."

I had heard his story many times, and this was my favorite part.

"I may have lost my previous life, but I gained eternal life. Now I look to Jesus because through him I can do anything. Well, almost anything. I'm still going to need those new wheels and a battery, Doc."

TODAY'S RX

You'll go further in life in the strength of the Lord.

Though my plans are not always the same as yours, Lord, I take comfort in knowing that your plans are best for me. Thank you for intervening in my life and keeping me close to you.

HEALING CAN BE A PROCESS

Jesus took the blind man by the hand and led him out of the village. Then, spitting on the man's eyes, he laid his hands on him and asked, "Can you see anything now?" The man looked around. "Yes," he said, "I see people, but I can't see them very clearly. They look like trees walking around." Then Jesus placed his hands on the man's eyes again, and his eyes were opened. His sight was completely restored, and he could see everything clearly.

MARK 8:23-25

Jesus could have healed the blind man completely on the first try. So why didn't he? The Gospel of John records a time when Jesus used saliva and mud to cure a blind man. Did he forget the secret mud ingredient this time? Did Jesus mess up?

We can become frustrated when things don't happen the way we want them to—or when we want them to. But I think Jesus did exactly what he intended to do. It's not that Jesus wasn't capable of healing the man instantly. Neither was it because the blind man had done anything wrong. Jesus healed the man the way he did because he wanted us to know something about his healing power.

Sometimes healing doesn't happen instantly. Sometimes healing is a process. I believe that Jesus didn't heal this man on the first try because he wanted to encourage us that even if all we get is a glimpse of the Lord's power, we shouldn't give up.

If your healing hasn't happened in the time, place, or way that you desired or hoped for, keep holding on to the hand of the Savior. Trust him to finish the good work he has started. Not every encounter with God allows us to see him clearly. Sometimes, all we see are blurry visions of "trees walking around." During those moments, it's important to remember that we shouldn't let go; we should continue to let God work.

Whether it is physical healing we're after or just trying to get a better glimpse of what God is doing in our lives, it may take more than one or two encounters before our sight is fully restored. Don't give up on the miracle that God wants to give you.

TODAY'S RX

If at first your prayers do not succeed, pray, pray again!

Lord, it's always in hindsight that I'm able to understand how you've worked in my life. Fill me with your Spirit today that I may trust your ways in the here and now, knowing you are with me wherever I go.

HEALING FAITH

A woman in the crowd had suffered for twelve
years with constant bleeding. She had suffered a
great deal from many doctors, and over the years
she had spent everything she had to pay them, but
she had gotten no better. In fact, she had gotten
worse. She had heard about Jesus, so she came
up behind him through the crowd and touched
his robe. For she thought to herself, "If I can just
touch his robe, I will be healed."

MARK 5:25-28

Lisa came to my office frustrated and exhausted. She
was out of money and out of hope.

"I've seen a dozen doctors, and no one has been
able to help me. They think I have some kind of
neurological problem, but all the tests come back
negative. I've used up all my insurance, and I'm
nearly broke. Can you help me?"

"I'm not sure I can do more than the other
doctors," I said. "But I can pray that God will reveal
the problem to us and lead us to a solution."

Looking at her chart, I understood why the other
doctors thought she was suffering from a seizure
disorder. Still, none of the treatments had worked.
Several tests had been repeated multiple times, with
inconclusive results. No wonder she was going broke!
I scratched my head and prayed. "Lord, help me
know where to search for an answer."

As only God would have it, I'd been talking

with a cardiologist recently about a new technology at the time—a thirty-day event monitor. I hoped that maybe this new technique would give us the information we needed to diagnose Lisa's mysterious ailment.

For two weeks, nothing happened, but on day fifteen, we captured the data we needed to diagnose a heart condition. Lisa had a pacemaker put in, and she's been doing fine ever since.

In today's verses, a woman who had tried every option and spent every resource in search of healing had only gotten worse. Still, when she heard about Jesus, she believed he could heal her if she could get close enough to touch his robe.

Is that the kind of faith we have? Too often, we take things into our own hands and turn to God only when nothing else works. What would happen if we turned to him *first*?

TODAY'S RX

To be healed, we must have the faith to reach out to Jesus.

Lord, help me to have faith in you. Whether I'm suffering physically, emotionally, or spiritually, show me that all I need is you. Thank you for your great healing power.

OUR GOD IS LARGE AND IN CHARGE

Why are you scheming against the LORD?
He will destroy you with one blow; he
won't need to strike twice!

NAHUM 1:9

Recently, I had to say farewell to one of my long-standing patients.

"Are you ready to be with Jesus?" I asked him when I knew his time was near.

His answer was an enthusiastic, "Yes! Yes! Yes!"

But his children were saying, "No, no, no. Lord, please don't take him," as they cried and mourned the loss that we all saw coming.

Once the patient had passed away and the family's tears slowed, they began to see his death with new eyes. They knew that one day in the future, their father would welcome them to their eternal home with great rejoicing. And on that day, their reunion would be complete.

Before the Fall, God's plan was for us to live with him in Eden, where we would never know disease or pain. But when sin entered the world, our physical lives were changed forever. Illness and sickness are God's enemies. And sometimes, they can seem like mighty enemies, scheming against us with pain and suffering.

God sent his son, Jesus, to reestablish the

covenant, and it is through our belief in Jesus that we know there is more to life than the physical life we see. Though Satan tries to destroy us, no plot or scheme of his can succeed against us. God promised us long ago that he will prevail and destroy the enemy with one blow.

When someone is sick, we pray for healing, and sometimes the Lord answers our prayers with a miraculous healing. But sometimes he doesn't. In such circumstances, we can feel as if the enemy has won. But God still heals us in death, as was the case with my patient. In death, God heals us with new bodies.

The glory of heaven can be hard to fully comprehend for those of us who are left behind. But what I can tell you from my experience sitting at the bedsides of so many dying saints is that both types of healing are answers to our prayers. And both are in God's sovereign will.

TODAY'S RX

Whether God heals us here and now or then and there, his answer to our prayer for healing is always "yes!"

Lord, let my heart be at peace with your will. However you choose to provide healing, may you ultimately be glorified.

GET TO KNOW HIM

The LORD is good to everyone. He showers
compassion on all his creation.

PSALM 145:9

"I've always lived my life on the edge," said Ray.
"That's why I don't expect I'll live to see sixty."

Ray was fifty-five years old, and he admitted to
smoking two packs of unfiltered cigarettes a day and
drinking a six-pack of beer every night. He'd also had
at least a couple of DUIs and spent time in jail for
use and possession of drugs. When he guessed that he
wouldn't live to see the age of sixty, it was probably
a good guess.

"Here's the deal," I replied. "Only God knows
the number of breaths and heartbeats we have left,
but you're facing some pretty serious health concerns.
Your lungs have been damaged with COPD—
chronic obstructive pulmonary disease—and your
chest X-ray shows a spot that may be cancerous.
I've set up an appointment for you to meet with a
pulmonary and thoracic surgeon next Monday."

By the following Thursday, Ray was in surgery,
and he returned to my rehab unit the week after that.
He seemed liked a different man. He was quieter and
showed less bravado.

"You know, Dr. Anderson, I've lived a terrible
life, and God is certainly going to punish me for
that," he said.

"Let me tell you something, Ray. You don't know God that well. He's not standing by with a sledgehammer, waiting to bash us. No, he showers us with grace. When we're lost and not even looking for him, he pursues us. He shines his blessings on all his creatures—good and bad. When we recognize his goodness and how he has extended his loving-kindness to us, it's natural to want to have a relationship with him. In fact, that's what happened to me many years ago. Had God not found me, I might be standing in your shoes. I just want you to know, it's not too late if you'd like to get to know him better."

"You're right. This cancer diagnosis scared me. When I get out of here, I'm going to church because I want to know him."

That was fifteen years ago, and Ray meant what he said. He just celebrated his seventieth birthday, and his life has become a blessing.

TODAY'S RX

You can't earn God's love, but you can yearn for God's love.

God, I need your grace each day. Thank you for continually pouring it out on me and for pursuing me with your everlasting love.

Day 33

NOTHING LASTS FOREVER... ESPECIALLY SUFFERING

In his kindness God called you to share in his
eternal glory by means of Christ Jesus. So after
you have suffered a little while, he will restore,
support, and strengthen you, and he will place
you on a firm foundation.

1 PETER 5:10

Tanya hadn't been on the schedule the last time I looked, so I was surprised to see her name penciled in as the last patient of the day. I knocked on the door and entered the exam room. When she saw me, she started to cry.

"What's going on?" I asked, sitting in the chair beside her. She looked tired and thin. "Why are you so sad?"

"I'm not sure I can take another day of this chemo/radiation treatment. I'm only on week three, and it already feels like forever. The oncologist says I need eight weeks, but I don't think I can make it that long. I'm sick and tired of feeling sick and tired."

"Can you tell me more about what's going on?"

"First thing every morning, I throw up everything I ate for dinner the night before. I feel horrible, but I can't go back to bed. I have to get in the car and drive forty-five minutes for another treatment. I've not only lost my hair, but I've lost my appetite. I feel like I've also lost my life!"

"What you're describing isn't unusual. Many people suffer similar side effects. I know it seems unbearable when you're in the middle of it. I've had other patients with the same kind of cancer and the same treatment, and they felt just like you do right now. But they kept fighting, and they made it through, and now they have their lives back."

"I guess I just needed to hear that there's hope, and that this will all be worth it."

"I know you can't see the end yet, but this treatment shows promise. Let's pray for strength and restoration for your body and your spirit."

Tanya and I prayed together, and she seemed reassured and committed to seeing the treatment through.

Suffering in any form is hard to take, but it helps to know that it won't last forever. Even in this broken world, our suffering is only for a little while.

TODAY'S RX
When life is hard, take one step at a time and watch for God's faithfulness in the journey.

Give me strength and energy today, God, to do all that is required of me. Help me to manage my stress and have a positive outlook on my work and responsibilities.

BE LIKE
THE OLIVE TREE

I am like an olive tree, thriving in the house
of God. I will always trust in God's unfailing love.

PSALM 52:8

Have you ever had the privilege of sitting under an olive tree? If you ever have the chance, I encourage you to soak up the experience.

When Karen and I visited the California wine country, we sat on a bench under an olive tree and had a picnic. It was a sunny afternoon, and the breeze that gently filtered through the branches cooled us. I watched as the sun's rays glistened on Karen's golden hair, making her look more radiant than ever. Sitting under the olive tree with my wife felt like a brief taste of heaven on earth.

As I breathed in the scent of olives all around me, I reflected on how important the olive tree has been to humanity. Throughout the centuries, the tree's branches have represented peace. After the Flood, the dove brought an olive branch back to Noah as the first evidence that man was once again reconciled with God.

The fruit of the olive tree has special healing properties that were well known in the ancient world and are being rediscovered in our day and age. We are beginning to realize that including olive oil in our diets can help prevent heart disease and hardening of the arteries. Some say that olive oil is one of the healthiest oils to cook with.

From the Old Testament, we learn how olive oil was used to fuel the lampstands in the Tabernacle. Jacob poured it on the stone pillar that he'd set up to mark the place where God had spoken to him. Olive oil was also used to anoint the sick, bake bread, and sanctify grain offerings.

No wonder the psalmist uses the olive tree as an image for thriving. The olive tree represents peace and calm, but also purpose and meaning. To live in the house of God as an olive tree would be an honor and a blessing that could be passed down for many generations. I pray for this for you as well as for myself.

TODAY'S RX

Whenever you use olive oil, remember its health benefits, along with how it was used in Old Testament times to glorify God.

Lord, help me to stand fruitful and pure, like an olive tree, in your sight. Use me to bring good news and light to others so that you may be glorified.

SEEING HIS ANSWER

Abraham never wavered in believing God's promise.
In fact, his faith grew stronger, and in this he
brought glory to God. He was fully convinced
that God is able to do whatever he promises.
And because of Abraham's faith, God counted
him as righteous. And when God counted him as
righteous, it wasn't just for Abraham's benefit. It was
recorded for our benefit, too, assuring us that God
will also count us as righteous if we believe in him,
the one who raised Jesus our Lord from the dead.

ROMANS 4:20-24

You've hoped and you've prayed. You've given and forgiven. You feel as if you've done everything God has asked of you, yet the disease still ravages your body unabated. In that dark moment, ask yourself a different question: What if God's answer to my prayer is not the same as what I'm asking for?

If God answers your prayers differently from how you want him to, does that mean prayer doesn't work? Do you give up on him?

God is the potter, and we are the clay. God molded us into being and breathed life into us. Without him, we would not be here to ask these questions.

Does the clay tell the potter that he isn't doing it right?

At first, Abraham doubted God's promise that he would become the father of nations. In fact, he doubted he would become the father of even one.

God eventually answered Abraham's prayer, but it wasn't how or when Abraham expected.

How would history be different if Abraham had stayed true to God's promises and hadn't had a son with Hagar? The conflict between the descendants of Abraham's two sons continues to this day.

Do we also risk future problems when we twist God's promises to fit our own desires? I know at times I've prayed for healing for my patients because that's what *I* wanted. Later, I discovered that their cancer had spread. Did God not answer my prayers?

Sometimes God's miraculous healing is to bring the patient's soul back to life, even as the body withers away. Is that not an answer to prayer?

Pray for God's will and not your own. Whatever answer comes, believe that it is God's complete and perfect will.

TODAY'S RX

God is faithful to answer our prayers, and his plan is perfect. Sometimes we have to adjust our expectations.

Help me to remain faithful to you, Lord, when my prayers seem unanswered. Do not let me fall away. I know all the days of my life are in your hand, and I take comfort in that.

HOLDING TIGHT
TO HOPE

Let us hold tightly without wavering to the hope we
affirm, for God can be trusted to keep his promise.

HEBREWS 10:23

I've had the privilege of escorting many of my patients
to heaven's front door. When I am with them during
their last moments on earth, the environment in
the room changes. A peace that surpasses all understanding enters the room, and a calm takes over. In
these moments, I know God is preparing to welcome
them to their forever home.

I witnessed this happen again recently.

I was at the hospital making my regular rounds,
and my next patient was in an adjacent building.
While walking down the enclosed corridor between
the buildings, I heard a code alert on the PA and
realized it was for my patient. I quickened my pace.

Marco was so ill that he appeared much older
than his forty-five years. His lungs were in such bad
condition from smoking that he had been on oxygen
for nearly a year. Yet, when the ambulance crew had
picked him up to bring him to the hospital, they
reported that he was smoking with his oxygen on.

We had tried everything we could to untangle
him from his addiction to tobacco but without
success. When I heard the code alert, I knew that his
lungs were likely failing for the last time.

I thought about the conversations we'd had over the past few years. He'd never been open to talking about his spiritual health—until last year. That's when he had accepted Jesus and started getting involved in his local church—as much as his health limitations would allow.

When I entered Marco's room, it was controlled chaos as the code team did its work. When they realized I was there, all eyes were on me for guidance.

I knew that Marco wanted us to try CPR, but he didn't want to be placed on life support. He was content with God's timing. After a short trial of CPR, we called time of death. As everyone else left the room, I lingered to feel God's presence. He had kept his promise to Marco to heal him for all eternity. Someday, he'll keep the same promise for us, as well.

TODAY'S RX

Make time today to record your end-of-life instructions. Decisions made in advance allow everyone there to be fully present in the moment.

I can only imagine how it must feel to be fully restored in body, mind, and spirit, Lord. Thank you for the promise of eternal life with you. Help me to sense your presence while I live out my time on earth and to draw near to you for your comforting embrace.

THE ENEMY IS CANCER

The eternal God is your refuge, and his everlasting
arms are under you. He drives out the enemy
before you; he cries out, "Destroy them!"
DEUTERONOMY 33:27

When we read today's verse, we know from its context that the armies fighting against the Israelites are the enemies that God drives out. Though this was written in Old Testament times, this verse is still applicable today. In my medical practice I hear God cry out, "Destroy them!" in a very different way.

Here's one example:

Bryant came in to get the results of a bone marrow test.

"The report confirmed our worst fear," I said. "I'm sorry to say . . . it's leukemia."

"But I was in six months ago, and all my blood work was normal."

"You're right. There was no hint of it at that time."

"So, how long have I had it?"

"It's hard to say. This is a fairly aggressive form of leukemia, but the good news is that we've caught it early on. I'll get an appointment for you to see the oncologist in the morning, and we will do what we can to defeat this enemy." Before he left, I promised to pray for him.

A week later, a letter from the oncologist confirmed what I had told Bryant. It was definitely leukemia, but being in an early phase made it treatable. The day after the oncologist examined him, Bryant started his treatment, and we all prayed for the best.

Six months later, Bryant stopped by my office.

"Great news, Dr. Anderson! The leukemia is in remission. And the oncologist is very hopeful."

We chatted about the good news, and before Bryant left, he said, "The Lord has given me new strength and new hope. Thank you for praying for me."

God hears our prayers, and he desires to drive out our enemies, even if they are unseen rogue cancer cells.

TODAY'S RX

Prayer can be the weapon that fights even the worst diagnosis. Remember, with God all things are possible—even driving out cancer.

Lord, you are the ultimate source of power and strength. Thank you for giving me courage to battle my illness. I look forward to when I stand victorious in your sight.

THE PAIN OF GROWING AND HEALING

I pray that your love will overflow more and more,
and that you will keep on growing in knowledge
and understanding.

PHILIPPIANS 1:9

"I don't know what's wrong with me," Gary said. He'd come to my office complaining of weight loss, night sweats, general malaise, and fatigue.

We did the usual in-office exam, and I didn't find anything remarkable. "Looking at your records, I see you were here about six months ago. Everything looked good then, and you were fit and healthy with no complaints. The only thing that's changed is you've lost fifteen pounds."

"Yeah, I'm kind of puzzled about that. I haven't been dieting."

Gary wasn't a smoker or a drinker, and he didn't have a family history that would indicate any problems. Without more clues to go on, the cause of his symptoms could be almost anything.

I ordered lab work and gave him the results a few days later. "It all came back negative, except for your white blood cell count. Yours was twenty-seven, which is about twice as high as normal. Your hematocrit was thirty, which is slightly low. I think I'll have you meet with a hematologist. He'll be able to run some specialized tests to see what's going on."

The next week, Gary was diagnosed with non-Hodgkin's lymphoma, an aggressive type of cancer that needed treatment. The specialist tried different chemotherapy treatments, but they all failed. Eventually, Gary's only option was to have a bone marrow transplant.

For the transplant to work, the treatment had to completely destroy Gary's existing bone marrow so his body wouldn't reject the donor marrow. It's a dangerous treatment primarily used in life-threatening situations. Fortunately, in Gary's case it worked.

Sometimes growth and healing involve rooting out or destroying something that isn't functioning properly for us. This is also true spiritually. If we want new life to grow, we must destroy old habits and destructive patterns of thinking.

The Bible refers to this as pruning the vine so that new life can develop and the vine can produce fruit. Is there something in your life that isn't functioning as it should? Whether it's an old habit or an old way of thinking, consider pruning the dead branches from your life as a way to help you grow stronger.

TODAY'S RX

Though pruning can be painful, the new growth will produce fruit that will make your pain a distant memory.

Lord, examine my heart. Please uproot and destroy the sinful behaviors that have taken hold and are spreading in my life. Replace them with your life-giving truth.

Day 39

GRANDMA'S HOPE, GOD'S MIRACLE

I pray that God, the source of hope, will fill you
completely with joy and peace because you trust in
him. Then you will overflow with confident hope
through the power of the Holy Spirit.

ROMANS 15:13

"I'm having pain in my right side," said Trina. "I have
indigestion and a lot of gas that seems to get worse
when I eat a fatty meal. What do you think is wrong?"

Trina was a classic gallbladder case. She presented
with the four *F*s we use to diagnose it: forty, fertile,
fat, and flatulent. Though her presentation was
textbook, something about her case seemed different.

I started by testing her gallbladder. The test
results showed a tumor in the pancreas, but it was
barely visible on the ultrasound. I ordered a CT scan,
which revealed that Trina had a large tumor covering
her abdomen. I sent her for consultations with
gastrointestinal and oncology surgeons, and they
both agreed: A Whipple procedure was Trina's only
hope; otherwise, she would have less than a year to
live. But the Whipple procedure wasn't a guarantee.
It is a complex operation that would remove parts
of her pancreas and small intestine, along with her
gallbladder.

When we met in my office to discuss her options,
Trina said, "I've prayed and prayed and decided to go

through with this. Not so much for me, but because I'm raising my two grandsons, and they need me to be here for them."

"Trina, I know this decision isn't easy, but I'm confident that God will honor your prayers. He will sustain you and fill you with peace, hope, and joy, even during the difficult days ahead."

Trina had surgery a few days later and came through without any problems—which, considering that her condition was much more complicated than originally diagnosed, was something of a miracle. From the initial diagnosis through a very complex surgery, God had heard and answered our prayers.

Four years later, not only has Grandma Trina been cured, but she is also filled with hope for the future as she watches her grandsons grow into the men God intended them to be.

My faith has been strengthened as well. I know that the Lord must have some mighty plans for those young men because he miraculously preserved Grandma Trina to raise them.

TODAY'S RX

God is able. With him, even the most difficult journey is possible.

Help me not to despair, Lord, when the road ahead is scary. I know you are able, and I trust that you will carry me through the heights and depths of this journey. Thank you for being near.

LOSING EVERYTHING BUT A PROMISE

As for me, I look to the LORD for help. I wait
confidently for God to save me, and my God
will certainly hear me. Do not gloat over me, my
enemies! For though I fall, I will rise again. Though
I sit in darkness, the LORD will be my light.

MICAH 7:7-8

Loretta was raised with money and manners, and
it showed in the way she held her head high and
walked with confidence. She was always dressed to
perfection and very well put together. But when her
husband of fifty-five years died, so did her elegance.
She seemed to lose her edge, and she cried a lot.

Her loss was monumental, and as time went on,
she began to lose weight and energy. We started her
on antidepressants, but she remained depressed. The
medication only slowed her downward spiral.

One busy day in my office, Loretta missed her
appointment. I made a mental note to call and
check on her when things slowed down, but before
I could phone her, I received a concerned call from
emergency medical services. Loretta had been found
on the floor at home, where she had lain for more
than fourteen hours before someone found her. That
alone could have been a terminal event, but even
more concerning was the result of the fall—a left
intertrochanteric hip fracture. To have the slightest

hope of recovery, Loretta would need surgery and extensive rehabilitation. I wasn't sure she had the emotional and mental fortitude it would require.

I prayed with her during this acute phase, and the Lord answered our prayers. Loretta made it through surgery and was transferred to the nursing home for rehabilitation. At first, her sadness continued, but eventually she started to get her old swing back. I knew things were headed in the right direction when she began putting on makeup before my scheduled visits to the home. Soon, the physical therapy department was praising her steps toward recovery. Three months later, she was back on her feet, and her smile was as radiant as ever.

"I'm proud of the progress you've made," I told her.

"Dr. Anderson, I lost everything, except for the promise that God would save me," she said. "And you know what? He did."

TODAY'S RX

When you fall, look up. God is there, and he has the power to heal and restore you.

God, help me to view my condition through your eyes— that it is temporary and that greater things are yet to come. Thank you for restoring my spirit.

THE GIVER OF LIFE IS ALSO THE GREAT HEALER

If you will listen carefully to the voice of the LORD
your God and do what is right in his sight, obeying
his commands and keeping all his decrees, then I
will not make you suffer any of the diseases I sent
on the Egyptians; for I am the LORD who heals you.

EXODUS 15:26

At the end of a long day, I entered John's room and
sat down beside his bed. He was asleep as I silently
prayed, *Please, God, don't let him die yet.*

John's wife and kids were all Christ followers, but
he had never seen a need for God. Now the acute
heart attack he'd had earlier that day was likely going
to be terminal.

Please, Lord, just a little more time, I prayed.

I thought about all the times when John had
visited my office. Though I'd known him for years, I
didn't know if he'd ever listened to my pleas to turn
his life around. It wouldn't have surprised me if he
hadn't. After all, he had never listened when I asked
him to quit smoking and drinking. I had also warned
him that the stress from his executive position was
taking a toll on his health. And now it appeared to
have worn out his heart.

As I finished my prayer and left the room, I
knew it might be the last time I'd see John. Only

the healing hand of God and the care of an excellent cardiac surgeon could save him now.

A few weeks later, I got a call from the cardiac rehab director. "I need to make a follow-up appointment for John."

Stunned, but elated that he'd made it through the surgery, I set up an appointment for the following week.

When John arrived at my office, I was prepared to have another hard conversation about his lifestyle with him. I also wanted to delve into the spiritual realm with him again. But he surprised me by introducing both topics first.

"The Lord spoke to me last night. And I'm ready to hear whatever wisdom you have for me."

John accomplished some amazing medical, physical, and lifestyle changes over the next few years. But the most astonishing change was how God had transformed him into a new creation.

TODAY'S RX

Show your appreciation for the gift of life by dedicating your days to the Giver of life.

Nothing is too challenging for you, Father. You soften the most stubborn hearts and bring people back to you. Thank you for softening my heart and allowing me to be your child.

GOD OF THE IMPOSSIBLE

Is anything too hard for the LORD? I will return
about this time next year, and Sarah will have a son.

GENESIS 18:14

Some things in life seem too hard even for the Lord
to do. In those moments we ask, "Is the God of the
impossible still with us? Can we still experience miracles like those found in the Old Testament?"

One day, a patient of mine named Bill asked me
to visit him at the hospital, where his wife, Carole,
was dying.

"The specialists say there's nothing they can do
for her," Bill said with tears in his eyes. "They said
it won't be long, and all we can do is wait for her
to die."

Across the room, Carole lay in bed, too weak
to talk. I watched her fight for every breath. The
surgeons had concluded that she was too weak for
surgery, and they recommended hospice care.

Hospice is designed to keep terminally ill patients
as comfortable as possible in their final days, to make
sure their health-care wishes are carried out, and that
they don't suffer needlessly. Patients typically leave
hospice only when they die.

I discussed Carole's final wishes with her and Bill.
She had a living will and a do-not-resuscitate order.
I knew that CPR would likely be painful and futile.
Before I left that night, the three of us prayed that

God would keep Carole alive so she would have more time with her family.

The next morning, I was surprised to hear that she was still alive. The day after that, she seemed a little better. A week later, her breathing was noticeably less labored and color had returned to her cheeks. I called a cardiovascular surgeon who was using some new, less-invasive techniques, and he agreed to see Carole.

Over the next few months, I received occasional updates from Bill as Carole made progress. A year later, at Bill's annual appointment, I was surprised to see a woman I barely recognized sitting with him. Carole's appearance had improved so much that she looked much younger than I remembered.

She glowed as she told me that she'd recently done something we all would have said was impossible a year earlier: "I danced with my son at his wedding!"

TODAY'S RX

Our God is still the God of the impossible. Pray with the knowledge that nothing you face is too big for him.

Father, I praise you that nothing is impossible in your sight. Thank you for working miracles to this day, and for giving me hope to continue persevering.

FREED FROM SIN AND BAD CHOICES

Because you belong to him, the power of the
life-giving Spirit has freed you from the power
of sin that leads to death.

ROMANS 8:2

When Adam and Eve chose to disobey God and eat
the forbidden fruit, they set the course of free, willful
disobedience that all of humankind would then
follow. As a result, sin entered the world and death
along with it. But we have hope because Jesus came
to rescue and redeem us from this broken world. All
we have to do is accept him as our Savior and put
our trust in him.

But even Jesus won't violate our free will.

Every day, I talk to patients who have a history of
making bad choices—whether it's smoking, excessive
drinking, overeating, lack of exercise, or illegal drug
use. In many cases, these choices have shortened their
natural lifespan by months, if not years.

When we turn away from our bad habits and
make good choices, sometimes the downward trend
of health problems can be slowed and occasionally
even reversed. If you're in such a situation, it's worth
the pain to change.

But even if we don't change our bad habits, we
can still change what happens when we sin. When
we turn to the Lord, he will release us from the

permanent death that is the wages for our sin. And that's a change worth making!

Though our physical bodies will one day fail us and return to dust, God has promised us eternal, heavenly bodies. These new bodies will be complete and healthy, free of sickness, disease, and weakness.

Jesus came to find me even when I wasn't looking for him. When he did, my life turned around 180 degrees from the way I was living before. Prior to meeting Jesus, I was on a pathway filled with sin, destruction, and death. Turning toward Jesus gave me a new life and lifted my spirit out of those destructive behaviors.

No matter which path you're currently on, I know that Jesus can rescue and redeem you. We were made to live perfectly in paradise, not stumbling sinfully through the world. But we have to choose Jesus if we want to be set back on track.

TODAY'S RX

It's not too late to change. Pick one bad habit today, and with the Lord's help, start making good choices.

Jesus, just as you redeemed this broken world, I thank you for how you'll one day fully redeem my body by making me a new creation in you. Thank you for overcoming sickness, weakness, and death and for continually making me new.

HE HEALED EVERY ONE

> After leaving the synagogue that day, Jesus
> went to Simon's home, where he found Simon's
> mother-in-law very sick with a high fever. "Please
> heal her," everyone begged. Standing at her bedside,
> he rebuked the fever, and it left her. And she got
> up at once and prepared a meal for them. As the
> sun went down that evening, people throughout
> the village brought sick family members to Jesus.
> No matter what their diseases were, the touch
> of his hand healed every one.
>
> LUKE 4:38-40

No matter what disease a person had, Jesus healed everyone! Even today, with our modern medical system, designer drugs, and technological tools, we cannot boast this kind of cure rate.

Many diseases still are considered incurable, and others have only a fifty-fifty chance of being cured. Even with the most established treatments, we don't always know who will respond and who won't. Sometimes, we have to try a second treatment option, or a third, because the first one failed to work.

For example, most infections are treated successfully today. But in Bible times, the simplest of infections could have had life-threatening consequences because antibiotics weren't yet available. While not always the case, some infections that cause a fever can resolve when the body's immune system kicks in. However, serious systemic infections can overcome the immune system, causing a toxic condition called *sepsis* and possibly resulting in death. But under the healing hands of Jesus, the viruses or bacteria were rebuked and ran for the hills, just like the demons did when Jesus commanded them to leave.

Today, we are learning that many of our "gold standard" treatments are failing because the disease microbes are developing a resistance to many anti-biotics. With Jesus, there was no resistance, only complete healing of every disease he encountered.

As a physician, I am increasingly in awe of our Lord's power, not only over the spiritual world but also over our physical world. I pray that his healing hands will touch you today and give you the strength and courage for your own healing journey.

TODAY'S RX

Even if you have been told you have a difficult case, remember, nothing is too difficult for Jesus. He alone can heal you completely.

God, I trust in you for complete healing for anything that comes my way. Help me to always be prayerful, thanking you for my health when I am well and seeking your strength when I am ill.

FAITH-BASED MEDICINE

Faith shows the reality of what we hope for; it is the
evidence of things we cannot see.
HEBREWS 11:1

When you visit the doctor and he or she outlines a treatment plan for your illness, you trust that the outcome will be what you expect. If the doctor says that this antibiotic will cure your sore throat, you take the pill and expect your throat to get better. But just as you put your trust in your doctor, doctors put their trust in their medical training and experience. Doctors don't just make up their treatment plans; they recommend a course based on what has been clinically proven to work for other patients.

We call this *evidence-based medicine*. Typically, the results of a study are reported as a percentage of positive results versus a percentage of negative results. Seventy percent positive is considered a great outcome. We'd like to have a 100 percent positive outcome, but that never happens. There are too many things we can't control that can cause treatments to fail. For example, an infection may develop resistance. Or one patient's body may not absorb the medication in the same way that someone else's body does, and thus the treatment won't be effective in all cases.

There's only one physician I know who can predict and produce a 100 percent positive outcome for everything he prescribes—the Great Physician.

So why don't we put our trust and faith in the good doctor who guarantees his treatment is 100 percent effective every time?

Some say it's because we can't see him.

That's not a problem for me. I have been at the bedsides of hundreds of dying patients over the years. And I have personally witnessed glimpses of heaven as many of them have crossed to the other side. I've watched God keep his promises. If you haven't personally seen the end result evidence and you wonder if it's prudent to place your trust in something you haven't seen, I remind you that we place our faith and trust in things we can't see all the time. For me, there is enough evidence that God keeps his promises that I will fully trust him until the day I die. I have faith in his faithfulness.

TODAY'S RX

The positive outcome for evidence-based medicine is 70 percent. Evidence-based salvation is 100 percent. If you haven't yet placed your faith in the Great Physician, do it today.

Father, I have faith in you to make me well. Thank you for guaranteeing me a home in heaven.

WHO GETS THE CREDIT?

When the Pharisees heard about the miracle, they
said, "No wonder he can cast out demons. He gets
his power from Satan, the prince of demons."

MATTHEW 12:24

When we look at today's verse, we might think, *Those
Pharisees! They don't understand that Jesus' healing
power comes from God the Father, not from Satan.*
We're quick to judge them because we know the end
of the story.

But are we really all that different from the
Pharisees?

In modern medicine, we often give credit to
doctors or researchers for their breakthroughs in
healing. We award the Nobel Prize for physiology
or medicine, but we don't give awards for healing
to the Great Physician. Shouldn't the credit for all
those award-winning insights or discoveries really go
to God?

In some cases, in their acceptance speeches,
the winners of the Nobel Prize thank God for his
guidance in their research and discoveries. However,
by the time the ceremony is over, the only name the
public remembers is the name of the person who
received the award, not the name of God.

Even in experimental scientific studies, we don't
account for God's hand in healing. When we study
new drugs or treatments, we compare them to a

placebo, which should have no scientific effect on the illness or disease. For a drug to receive approval from the Food and Drug Administration, it must be statistically better than a placebo. That makes sense. An effective treatment should be better than something that is supposed to do nothing.

But what if a placebo isn't actually doing nothing? What if, in some cases, the placebo is actually the means by which God does his healing? Every year, there are thousands of drugs and treatments studied by scientists or doctors that don't do any better than the placebo. And study after study reveals that placebos can have measurable cure rates. In other words, doing something that should have no scientific reason to affect a cure often does.

I believe this is evidence that we are like the Pharisees. We don't give credit to God for the cure when he is ultimately the source of all healing.

TODAY'S RX

Give credit where credit is due. Don't overlook the hand of God in your healing.

Lord, please forgive me for when I've doubted you or turned a blind eye to you. You are the healer of all. Even when I am struggling or in pain, help me to always acknowledge your faithfulness.

TURN OFF TECHNOLOGY TO TURN OFF ANXIETY

The LORD himself will fight for you. Just stay calm.

EXODUS 14:14

Regina came to me with a series of complaints. "I don't know what's going on. My heart is racing, my hands are sweating, and there are times when I can't get a good breath."

I asked her some questions and ordered a few tests. Over the next week, we ruled out a range of possible causes, including problems with her heart or lungs, a stroke, and thyroid disease. Yet her symptoms persisted—which is what eventually confirmed my diagnosis.

"Regina, the tests show you're in great physical shape. All of your results were normal. I'm pretty sure what's causing your symptoms is generalized anxiety disorder, caused by the stress you're under."

Of course, the diagnosis did what I expected it would—it raised her anxiety level.

Anxiety is one of the more common diagnoses in America—some might call it an epidemic. I see it on a daily basis with my patients.

"What do I do about it?" Regina asked. "I'm already stressed enough. I can't keep feeling this way."

"The best thing you can do is avoid the things that cause anxiety. For example, if the news upsets you, stop reading the headlines and watching TV.

Take a few hours a day to step away from technology. Put your phone in another room, and turn off the TV and the computer. We were created to live in a garden, not in a world overflowing with bits and bytes. No wonder our brains are screaming for peace and tranquility."

"But am I supposed to just stare at the walls during that time?"

"Use it as a time to reconnect with your friends, family, and God. Go outside and take a walk. Keep a journal about the things you're thinking and feeling. Use the time to pursue things you enjoy."

"That does sound more relaxing, but I'm constantly fighting deadlines at work, and I need my computer."

"Ultimately, if you're not as anxious, you'll make better use of technology. Your brain will work better because you'll be worrying less."

TODAY'S RX

Sometimes, in order to keep calm, we must unplug and just relax.

Lord, I confess that I'm often so distracted by all the day's demands that I do not spend regular quiet time with you. Help me to create space in my day to read your Word and pray. Thank you for the renewal I feel when I invest time with you.

FAITH TO HEAL WITH SPIT, MUD, OR JUST PLAIN WORDS

He spit on the ground, made mud with the saliva,
and spread the mud over the blind man's eyes. He
told him, "Go wash yourself in the pool of Siloam"
(Siloam means "sent"). So the man went and
washed and came back seeing!

JOHN 9:6-7

If a man complained to you that he had something in his eye and couldn't see, what would you do to help him? You might take a look to see if you could remove whatever was obstructing his vision. Or maybe you'd help him flush his eye with water.

Chances are good that you wouldn't say, "Hold still while I spit on the ground, make some mud with my saliva, and apply it to your eyes. That'll fix you right up!" Yet that's exactly what Jesus did.

This seems like such a crazy thing for him to do. In so many other cases when he healed people, either he reached out and touched them, or he simply healed them with a word. But in this case, Jesus used two very unlikely, and very unlovely, things to help the man see.

When analyzed chemically, both mud and spit have some medicinal properties. Saliva comes from one of the more bacteria-infested areas of the body. Its purpose is to sterilize the dirty food (and sometimes even dirt itself) that finds its way into our mouths. The enzymes in our saliva begin to break down the food, disrupting the cells of the bacteria.

If the man's blindness were due to something on the surface of his corneas, it might make sense to utilize the abrasive properties of mud by rubbing it on his eyes. As doctors, we often must debride diseased tissue from an area before we will see new and healthy growth. That's essentially what laser procedures do, and we use them all the time for treatment of various eye conditions.

Jesus knew exactly what this man needed and treated him with the most appropriate—though unlikely—elements. But the healing was no less miraculous. We could not simply repeat his actions and expect the same outcome, but we can be certain that Jesus could have healed the man's eyes with a word—and that the same healing is available to us.

TODAY'S RX

Consider that Jesus may use unusual methods, tools, or people to heal you.

Father, your power is made perfect in our weakness, and you continue to show that power in numerous ways. Thank you for healing our sicknesses and disabilities through whatever means necessary.

RESCUED FROM FAMINE

The LORD watches over those who fear him, those
who rely on his unfailing love. He rescues them
from death and keeps them alive in times of famine.

PSALM 33:18-19

Caroline came into my office for a follow-up visit,
but her cough hadn't gotten any better.

"You look like you've lost weight," I said.

"With the fever, I haven't been hungry," she said.

"You know the saying, 'Feed a cold, starve a
fever'?" I said. "That's wrong. It should be 'Feed a
cold, feed a fever.'"

"Okay, I'll try to eat more," she said.

"Did you take what I prescribed for the
bronchitis?" I asked.

"Every day, just like you said."

A fever can help our bodies beat an infection, but
after several courses of antibiotics, Caroline's fever
was past that point.

"I'm going to order a chest X-ray. Your cough
should be better by now."

When the results came back, I noticed a spot
in the region of the chest cavity that contains all
the chest organs except the lungs. Further testing
confirmed our worst fear: Caroline had lung cancer.
Unfortunately, it was located in a spot that surgery
couldn't get to. Her only hope was chemotherapy.
With her already depressed immune system, I knew

it would be a difficult journey—and the chemo beat her up pretty badly. She lost even more weight, and her once-beautiful hair fell out.

Three months after the chemo ended, Caroline arrived for a follow-up visit, sporting a baseball cap. Tests showed that the tumor had shrunk by 70 percent, but it was now at a standstill, and there was nothing more we could do. Caroline and I agreed that we would continue to pray for remission.

Then I noticed something else in her chart. "Have you gained five pounds?" I said. No one gains weight while on chemo.

Caroline grinned. "Yes, Dr. Anderson. I figured if eating could help me beat a cold, it might also help me beat this cancer!"

Caroline experienced a famine on a personal level, and yet God had kept her alive. Her story is a reminder to me of how God's ancient promises are still applicable today.

TODAY'S RX

Keep eating and drinking when you're sick. Proper nutrition and hydration help your body fight disease.

God, rescue me from all that plagues my mind and body. Nourish me with your promises, and strengthen my spirit with your Word.

SURPRISING WORDS

Stretch out your hand with healing power; may
miraculous signs and wonders be done through
the name of your holy servant Jesus.

ACTS 4:30

During an overnight shift in the ER, I was summoned
to see a young boy who had fallen and hit his head.

"I heard that throwing up after hitting your head
is a bad thing, so I brought him in," his mother said.

Though it was 1:30 in the morning, the mother
was fully dressed and completely made up. *If she had
time to get ready, how serious could it be?* I wondered
as I started my exam.

The boy's pupils were equal and reactive. He was
attentive and easily followed my directions. "Where
did you hurt your head?" I asked. He pointed to the
spot, and I felt it.

It was a normal neural exam. He was a normal
kid who'd gotten a bump on the head. But as I turned
to ask the nurse to give the mother a head injury
instruction sheet, I heard myself say instead, "Well,
his exam looks good, but I think we should send him
to Vanderbilt to get a CT scan."

I had no idea why I'd said that. The words just
slipped out of my mouth. The nurse looked at me
like I was a lunatic, and the mother seemed confused.
Without knowing why, I sensed that something more
was going on.

It was no small thing to find a neurosurgeon in the middle of the night. Moreover, the nurse had to order an ambulance to take the boy, and there was a ton of paperwork involved.

Though I had no objective data to back up my referral, I had a sense that something was happening that only God could explain.

Four hours later, the neurosurgeon phoned and surprised me with these words: "I'm glad you sent him over. I just got out of surgery. We evacuated a hematoma from his brain. If you hadn't gotten him here in time, he would have died."

I'm convinced that it was God who spoke the words to send that boy to Vanderbilt; he simply used my mouth to do it.

TODAY'S RX

When you hear a still, small voice, be open to it. You just might witness a miracle.

Father, I invite you to speak through me today, offering kindness and counsel to those around me who are in need. May my words be pleasing to you and a comfort to those who are hurting.

SOUL SURVIVOR

Now may our Lord Jesus Christ himself and
God our Father, who loved us and by his grace
gave us eternal comfort and a wonderful hope,
comfort you and strengthen you in every
good thing you do and say.

2 THESSALONIANS 2:16-17

Trey's journey had been most unusual. As I sat down next to him, he began to tell me about it.

"When I was fifteen," he said, "I got drunk and high one night. I was supposed to meet a girl at the crossroads of the main highway and the railroad tracks that ran through town. But she wasn't there, so I just sat down to wait for her. I didn't realize I was sitting in the middle of the train tracks. That's obviously not a smart thing to do, but at the time, I was drunk and high and not thinking clearly."

Trey paused and looked off into the distance, as if remembering something.

"The next thing I remember hearing was the screech of a train. It was as if time stood still in that moment. A light that was so bright surrounded me, and I couldn't see anything else. Then this lone figure approached. It was a man, and he reached out for me. It was my grandfather, and he was asking me if I was ready to go with him."

But Trey's grandfather had died ten years earlier.

"I didn't feel anything when the train hit me. It

wasn't until six months later, when I woke up in the ICU with the right side of my skull crushed, that I felt anything at all. I almost died twice."

"What do you mean you almost died twice?" I asked.

The day I woke up was the same day my parents had agreed to remove me from life support. But somehow, Jesus protected me and helped me."

"Wow, that's quite a journey, Trey. How did it change your life?"

"Without a doubt, I knew that it was Jesus who gave me the strength to overcome my injuries. He's been my comfort every day for thirty-five years since it happened. Each day, I wake up looking for him, and he's always right there by me—just like he was when I spent those six months in a coma."

TODAY'S RX

No matter how bad the train wreck, God can put your life back on track.

Father, you are my wonderful hope. Thank you for rescuing me in times of trouble.

JOB-RELATED BENEFITS OF TAKING CHRIST TO WORK

They began their circuit of the villages, preaching
the Good News and healing the sick.

LUKE 9:6

When I moved to Cheatham County, I was the third
doctor in the county. Though I knew that at least one
of the other two doctors was a believer, I also knew
that he believed it was best to separate his faith from
his work. That made me the only openly Christian
doctor practicing in that rural community.

For me, the decision to be both a Christian
and a Christian doctor was an easy one. Though
it seemed that some people were able to put their
faith and their work into separate boxes, God had
always jumbled my boxes together. There was no way
I could function as a doctor without God's backing
or leading.

So often in today's world, we live our Christian
lives apart from everything else we do. We don't want
to be perceived as ignorant and politically incorrect
or narrow-minded. But in my experience, following
Jesus is the most politically correct and open-minded
thing we could ever do. Jesus taught us to love one
another. And he taught us to win others to faith
through our love for them and each other. My faith
doesn't make me intolerant, it makes me more loving.

I have never met a patient for whom I didn't wish the best, regardless of what his or her beliefs were.

As Christians, our position is one of serving and pointing the way to God. Just as the gospel and healing went hand in hand in today's verse—in fact, in the whole New Testament—I've learned they go hand in hand in my office too. Years of practicing medicine as an openly Christian doctor have given me the opportunity to share my faith in ways that encourage others who are experiencing the greatest hurts this broken world has to offer. I've received countless invitations to be with families and be a part of their conversations during their most trying hours. Being asked to pray with and for a patient in one of those situations is one of the greatest gifts of living an openly Christian lifestyle at work.

TODAY'S RX

Love others so much today that tomorrow they will invite you into their lives and share their hurts.

Father, help me to proclaim your name through all I do and say. May I point others to your love by serving them well and helping them through their hurts.

TEENAGE TEARS

Let your unfailing love comfort me, just
as you promised me, your servant. Surround
me with your tender mercies so I may live,
for your instructions are my delight.

PSALM 119:76-77

"Courtney has lost a lot of weight," her mom said,
"and I am worried about her. Can you run some tests
to see what's wrong?"

Courtney sat on the exam table picking at her
nails, looking down the entire time her mother spoke.
I'd taken care of Courtney since she was an infant. I'd
watched her grow into a kind and generous young
woman. But something wasn't right. She wasn't her
usual bubbly self.

"May I speak with Courtney privately?" I said.

Her mother agreed to give us some space and
stepped out of the room.

I knew this would be a hard conversation to have
with a seventeen-year-old, but I hoped she knew me
well enough to feel comfortable telling me what was
really going on.

"Courtney, the last time I saw you, you weighed
150 pounds, and now you're down to 120. Why do
you think you're losing weight?"

"I guess it's because I'm not eating very well. I
hide it. I tell my family that I've already eaten or that

I'm going to go out to eat with friends, but then I never do."

"Why is that?"

"I don't know. I guess I'm not hungry."

"How are you sleeping?"

"Not good. Ever since I broke up with my boyfriend, I can't fall asleep. I wake up in the middle of the night and just lie there thinking or crying."

"Tell me about that."

"I thought Josh and I were going to get married when we graduated. But now . . . I don't know what I'm going to do."

If anyone you know is having trouble with sleep or appetite, look to see if there's an emotional cause. This can often point the way to a diagnosis. Fortunately, for Courtney, things got better. A few months after our appointment, she had regained her confidence. And not long after that, another boy asked her to the homecoming dance.

As adults, our job is to guide our teens and encourage them to seek Jesus as their source of confidence.

TODAY'S RX

Tears and the teen years commonly go together. But if the tears reach flood stage, look for professional help.

Father, may I be a source of encouragement and light to the teens in my life. Help me to plant seeds of faith in their lives and show them that they have worth.

WHO ELSE?

That evening many demon-possessed people
were brought to Jesus. He cast out the evil spirits
with a simple command, and he healed all the sick.
This fulfilled the word of the Lord through the
prophet Isaiah, who said, "He took our sicknesses
and removed our diseases."

MATTHEW 8:16-17

This story of Jesus taking our physical illness and removing our diseases is just a foreshadowing of greater things to come. On the cross, not only did Jesus take our sicknesses, he also took all of the sins of the world—past, present, and future. His death made us clean and spiritually healthy once again.

No matter how hard we try, and even with all of the tools of modern medicine, doctors cannot heal everyone. Even diseases that have cure rates nearing 100 percent still have isolated cases that don't respond to treatment. But with Jesus, his cure rate is always 100 percent.

When we look to Jesus for healing, we need to understand that his healing isn't limited to just our earthly world. Sometimes, to see his healing hands at work, we need to look beyond this world and realize that he may heal something greater than just our mortal bodies. He may choose not to heal us here on earth; he may want us to wait until he heals us permanently, for all of eternity.

Who else but Jesus could take our illnesses and heal them by the touch of his hand? Who else but Jesus and his death on the cross could heal our mortality?

The answers we receive to our prayers and requests for healing may be different from what we are asking, but that doesn't mean God hasn't heard or that he has denied us healing. Healing can occur on both sides of the veil that separates this world from the next. Complete healing of our mortal bodies will only happen on the other side of the veil.

TODAY'S RX

Look expectantly for God's healing, wherever it may happen.

Father, give me the courage to accept your plan for me, even when it deviates from what I ask. Embolden my faith so that I may trust you with all my heart through whatever lies ahead.

HEALING HANDS

Be strong and immovable. Always work
enthusiastically for the Lord, for you know that
nothing you do for the Lord is ever useless.
1 CORINTHIANS 15:58

In medical school, we were taught that if we listened to our patients, they would give us their diagnosis. When a doctor touches a patient, I believe he or she receives confirmation of what the patient has expressed in words. I often find myself "listening" with my hands so I can feel what my patient feels. I believe that God gave me a gift, similar to a mother's sensitivity to her child's pain or illness, which has been sharpened through my medical training and practice.

When I am examining a patient with my hands and come across sudden warmth, I know something may be awry. When that happens, I start my search for a diagnosis where my hands felt the warmest. Often, it leads me to diseases I might not otherwise have considered. Patients seem to appreciate my high-touch diagnostic skills, and the more I use them, the more I recognize them as a God-given gift.

God has given you certain gifts and talents as well. Maybe it's an ear for music, a heart for hospitality, or a special ability to relate to children or teenagers. Whatever it is, know that it is not merely a gift from God to you. It is a gift from God *through* you to those around you—a way for you to serve and bless others and use your talent for God's glory.

When we get to heaven, we will be exactly who God created us to be, minus the burden of sin and worldly concerns. We will freely do, to the fullest extent, what God created us to do. Here in this life, the deep joy and satisfaction we feel whenever we are faithful stewards of God's gifts is just a tiny foretaste of what awaits us in our heavenly home.

TODAY'S RX

Ask God what he wants you to do with the talents he has given you. If you feel as if you're not using your gifts to the fullest extent, what is holding you back?

God, thank you for the gifts you have given me. I know that any talents or abilities I have are not from my own doing, but are from you. Help me to use these gifts well so that I may point others to you.

Day 56

EXPECT A MIRACLE,
TELL THE STORY

If God is for us, who can ever be against us?

ROMANS 8:31

If you saw Norm sitting in my waiting room, he wouldn't look any different from any of the other blue-collar workers waiting to see me. He wore flannel work shirts and dungarees and drove an old Ford pickup, but Norm wasn't part of the crew—he was the guy who owned the company.

I didn't know how much money he made, but I knew he had riches beyond this world that he valued more than anything.

Norm entered the exam room and sat down in a chair instead of on the examining table. "Dr. Anderson, I've been pretty vocal about my faith for a long time, but after what I've been through recently, I have even more reason to talk about it."

I had always known Norm to be outspoken about his faith. He'd once brought me a sign that said, "Without God, there is no America."

"When I turned seventy, I went in for my screening like you said. Well, the doctor told me I had a triple A, which sounded like a good grade to me but turned out to be bad news—an abdominal aortic aneurysm, which can be really dangerous. I told the surgeon, 'If it's my time to go, I'm going to go.' But he talked me into doing the surgery anyway."

"That's a pretty big operation, even for someone young and healthy," I said.

"I know," he said. "The surgeon said that all was going well, but then my kidneys started to fail and so did my heart. Turns out I nearly died in surgery, and they had to take me to the ICU. But that wasn't the only thing that happened. During that time, I saw Jesus. He turned me around and told me I had to go back, that I had more work to do here on earth. And he wasn't talking about my business; he was talking about doing *his* business. So now that I'm back, I'm telling everyone who will listen."

Norm told me that he'd come home from the hospital and rehab six weeks earlier than anyone expected. "Do you believe in miracles, Doc? Because I sure do!"

TODAY'S RX

Trust in the Lord and expect a miracle. Then, like Norm, tell everyone about it.

Jesus, help me to share my faith with others, offering them the same life-giving hope that you offered me. May their ears be open to your story, and may their lives be changed.

PRAYING FOR A SHOT TO SING

My heart is confident in you, O God; no wonder
I can sing your praises with all my heart!

PSALM 108:1

Nashville is affectionately called Music City, and it seems there is a venue for live music on nearly every corner. Musicians and wannabes flock to Nashville to work in the industry, or at least to rub shoulders with like-minded individuals.

Many of my patients are in the music business, and those who sing depend on their voices to make a living. Unlike a piano player, for example, when vocalists get sick, they can literally lose their jobs, so it puts a lot of pressure on me when they can't sing.

Toni came to see me in the middle of flu season. It seemed that nearly every patient I saw that week had some sort of upper respiratory ailment.

"I can't talk, much less sing," she whispered. "And I have an audition tomorrow. I've been working on it for months, and I really need the job."

She looked pitiful sitting on the exam table. Her eyes were droopy, and her cheeks were flushed. She could barely speak above a whisper.

I ran some tests, and the results weren't good. She had both strep and mono. Either one would be difficult to cure in time for her audition the next day, but with both, it was next to impossible. But together we would do what we could. I gave her a shot of antibiotics for the strep and a steroid shot to shrink the lymph tissue. That seemed like the best option considering the importance of her audition.

"This will get things started, but I need you to come back and see me next week, so I can make sure you're recovering."

"Of course!" she whispered. "But can you also pray for my audition? I really need this gig . . ."

I took her hands in mine, and we prayed for healing and for God's will to be done at her audition.

The next week, Toni came back to the office. Not only did she feel better, but she was full of thanks and praise to Jesus.

"I got the tour!" she said, her voice as strong as ever. "I think the shots helped, but the prayers helped even more."

TODAY'S RX

Even when it seems like a shot in the dark—pray!

Whenever I'm too lazy to pray, Lord, remind me that it is my lifeblood—that it keeps me hopeful and in communication with you for all that I need. Thank you for never being too lazy to listen.

Day 58

THE POWER IS HIS

I also pray that you will understand the incredible
greatness of God's power for us who believe him.
This is the same mighty power that raised Christ
from the dead and seated him in the place of honor
at God's right hand in the heavenly realms.

EPHESIANS 1:19-20

"Tell me what's going on," I said to Erin. It had been
a while since her last appointment.

"Oh, I'm not having any problems. I just haven't
had a checkup in a while, and I thought I should
probably get one."

"Great, I'm glad you're feeling well." As I glanced
at her paperwork, something caught my eye. "Looks
like you marked "yes" to both abdominal pain and
recent weight loss. Tell me more about that."

"Oh, I just marked it because it asked, but I'm
not really having any problems," she said.

I asked Erin more specific questions about her
pain and the amount of her weight loss, but she
assured me it was nothing.

"There are a couple of things that concern me," I
said. "I think we should have them checked out just
to make sure."

The following week, I sat at my desk staring
in disbelief at Erin's test results. They showed a
metastatic renal cell carcinoma—cancer of the
kidneys that had spread to other organs.

When I gave Erin the diagnosis, her eyes filled with tears as she tried to understand how she could go from feeling good to being diagnosed with an incurable illness.

I took her hand and said, "Only the Lord knows our time on earth and the journey he has ordained for us to travel. As your doctor, I promise to do everything I can to make your journey as pain-free and comfortable as possible. As your friend and brother in Christ, I will continue to pray for God's healing hand and mercy upon you."

Though I look forward expectantly to one day crossing from this world to the next, I know that many people are not prepared to face the end of their time here on earth—certainly not before they might expect it. My best advice is to prepare your heart and soul for eternity before you are confronted with the reality of your mortality. Above all, trust God. Only he knows when your day will arrive.

TODAY'S RX

God holds the power of life and death. Entrust him with your destiny.

Plant a desire for heaven deeper in my heart, Lord. Help me to realize how temporary my time on earth is, and allow me to use the days I have left in a way that brings you glory.

A SAVIOR AMID
THE CORNSTALKS

He lifted me out of the pit of despair, out of the
mud and the mire. He set my feet on solid ground
and steadied me as I walked along.

PSALM 40:2

I was ten weeks into a twelve-week summer job selling
the Volume Library door-to-door in southern Illinois.
As I drove past towering cornfields, I rehearsed my
next house call, where I hoped to find an eager buyer.
Instead of paying attention to the road, I was studying
the map and my notes on the passenger seat.

Then it was too late.

An eighteen-wheeler sideswiped my Volkswagen
Beetle, tossing my Bug up and onto the grille of the
truck, where I became a hood ornament. When the
semi finally came to a stop a hundred yards from
where we first made contact and once my brain
stopped swimming, I looked up to see the truck
driver staring at me, white as a ghost.

He jumped out, ran toward me, and managed
to pry open my crumpled door, using some kind of
superhuman strength.

"Son, I didn't see you. Are you all right?"

His words echoed in my head until I understood
what he was asking. "I think so," I said. I felt a little
woozy, but otherwise I was fine. A tear rolled down my
cheek as I realized I had just been spared a tragic death.

"I'll go get help," the driver said as he staggered back to his rig.

By the time he got back, my mind and heart had settled a bit. Though at the time I professed to be an atheist, somewhere inside I knew that God was the one who had spared my life. He alone knew my past and where my heart was at that moment. Instead of allowing me to die, alone and apart from him, he picked me up and set me back on solid ground. Three years later, when he revealed himself to me in a dream, I was ready to turn back to him.

Today, I look back at the accident and my second chance, and I thank God for being there and caring for me, even when I didn't care to know him. I believe he saved me that day to give me time to come back to him.

TODAY'S RX

God can change the direction of your life at any given moment—but it's less painful if you turn to him first.

God, help me to realize day in and day out how you intervene in my life to keep me from harm's way. May I have a thankful heart, knowing that you are my protector.

HIDDEN HURTS

He heals the brokenhearted and
bandages their wounds.
PSALM 147:3

When I make rounds, the nurses will update me on any changes with my patients. Typically this means vital signs, inputs and outputs (I/Os), and how many bandage changes on wounds.

More experienced nurses will often give me insight into a patient's anger or depression or tell me about a visitor who was especially upsetting. Many times, the patients themselves will tell me when there's more going on than meets the eye.

Through the years, I've learned a lot about my patients while dressing wounds, casting broken bones, or waiting for X-rays to come back. During those times, patients may open up a bit and share the story behind the story that brought them to the hospital. The physical injury becomes the beginning of an invitation to hear about what's really hurting them.

Amy's ankle injury was not particularly severe, but the story of how the injury occurred brought a whole new level of concern. She had fallen down a set of stairs and twisted her ankle on the landing—but then she told me she'd been pushed down the stairs while being kicked out of her house. Once we got her patched up, she began to cry that she had nowhere to go.

We made a few phone calls and found a women's shelter where she would be safe and have a roof over her head.

Amy's ankle healed slowly, along with her broken heart. Eventually, she found a new home and a job. With independence came a new sense of confidence that transformed the timid, frightened young woman I had first met in the ER.

Though Amy had been injured in her fall down the stairs, I saw it as God's intervention to protect her from greater harm, while he simultaneously pushed open a door that Amy had desperately tried to keep shut—bringing healing to the root of her problem.

Sometimes it can seem as if no one sees or cares about your pain. In those moments, be still and know that God not only cares for your bumps and bruises, he also cares for your banged-up and bruised heart. He has the power and the compassion to heal them both.

TODAY'S RX

Whether others see your pain or not, be assured that the Great Physician sees everything, and he has a treatment plan to restore you to health, inside and out.

Father, thank you for tending to my heart. Even when all seems lost and I feel alone, I have the promise of your presence beside me, caring for me and walking me toward healing.

HEALING FLOWS FROM GOD

Fruit trees of all kinds will grow along both sides
of the river. The leaves of these trees will never
turn brown and fall, and there will always be
fruit on their branches. There will be a new crop
every month, for they are watered by the river
flowing from the Temple. The fruit will be for
food and the leaves for healing.

EZEKIEL 47:12

Ezekiel was an Old Testament prophet who had an apocalyptic vision of the Temple, God's dwelling place, metaphorically revealed to be the source of divine, life-giving water.

This reminds me of the Amazon River and the surrounding rain forests. Did you know that many of our favorite foods, such as oranges, lemons, grapefruits, figs, bananas, pineapples, coconuts, and mangoes are found in the rain forest? Though in the West we eat only about two hundred different kinds of fruit, natives of the area have access to a much broader diet, including nearly two thousand varieties of fruit.

Rain forest plants are also rich in medicinal properties. Nearly one out of every four ingredients in our modern medicines comes from the flora grown there. Furthermore, two thousand plants found in the rain forest have proven anticancer properties. It's as if the rain forest is nature's pharmacy, providing us with healthy foods and healing medicine.

It's exciting when scientists discover new technological breakthroughs in food and medicine. But we must remember that some of the greatest modern miracles were discovered in trees and shrubs that God gave us thousands of years ago. Healing can come to us in many forms. Sometimes it comes miraculously. Other times it comes through medicine, and still other times it happens through healthy eating choices.

As today's verse mentions, a river flowed from the Temple with healing waters, which nourished the trees on both sides. The trees were also a source of food and medicine. Ezekiel poetically reminds us that no matter how we're healed, healing always flows from God.

TODAY'S RX

The healing properties of food aren't found in a vending machine. If you can grow it or pick it, you'll be much closer to the way God intended you to eat.

Lord, I desire to fill my body with the healthy, nourishing foods you intended for me to eat—not the sugary, processed foods that lack nutritional value. Help me to make wise choices to keep my body running well.

PLANS TO PROSPER

"I know the plans I have for you," says the LORD.
"They are plans for good and not for disaster,
to give you a future and a hope."
JEREMIAH 29:11

I hadn't seen Bert, or any members of his family, for more than three years. Then he showed up one day with a form for me to sign.

"I need to have a physical for my new job," Bert said. "I'm hoping everything checks out because it's been a while since I was last here."

"It has been a long time, hasn't it?" I said, looking at his chart.

"The downturn in the economy just about did us in. We had to sell our house and rent an apartment in the low-rent section of town. I need this job. I've got to get my kids out of there and move them to a better school district."

"Bert, I know this job is very important to you and to your family. And I know you've tasted bitter waters and survived up to this point, though I'm sure sometimes it didn't seem like you would. But I want you to know that regardless of what this exam shows, I am confident that God has a good plan for you and for the life of your family."

I thought about the above verse in Jeremiah and prayed that God would deliver on that promise for Bert.

During his exam, a couple of small things revealed themselves, but they were minor problems. Frankly, they were the kinds of stress-related, wear-and-tear issues I'd expect to see on anyone who'd been through what he and his family had been through for the past three years.

"There's nothing in this exam that will keep you from getting the job," I said. I happily signed his form.

"I promise once my new insurance kicks in, I will get the kids here for their well visits and their shots. I can't tell you how blessed I am that God carried us through those dark times." Bert was whistling as he walked out the door.

I wish all my patients would believe what Bert already knew to be true. God's plans are never meant to harm or hurt us. His plans are always for our good.

TODAY'S RX

Even in our darkest hours, our heavenly Father shines his light to show us the way to the fulfillment of his promises.

Though my future is unclear, Lord, I know you are in control. Help me not to rely on my own strength and understanding, but to depend on you to lead me to pathways of healing and light.

HEALTHY PEOPLE DON'T NEED A DOCTOR

As Jesus left the town, he saw a tax collector named
Levi sitting at his tax collector's booth. "Follow me
and be my disciple," Jesus said to him. So Levi got
up, left everything, and followed him. Later, Levi
held a banquet in his home with Jesus as the guest of
honor. Many of Levi's fellow tax collectors and other
guests also ate with them. But the Pharisees and their
teachers of religious law complained bitterly to Jesus'
disciples, "Why do you eat and drink with such
scum?" Jesus answered them, "Healthy people don't
need a doctor—sick people do. I have come to call
not those who think they are righteous, but those
who know they are sinners and need to repent."

LUKE 5:27-32

As a family care physician, I often do annual physical
exams on my healthy patients. Sometimes they just
want to make sure everything is okay. Other times,
they need a physical for sports, school, a new job,
or to qualify for insurance. If I declare them free of
illness, they walk away happy—and I'm happy for
them; but I find these encounters to be less fulfilling
than working with patients who are sick or dying. My
job, training, and experience are all about helping the
sick and suffering. The more time I spend with my
well patients or my worried-they-might-not-be-well
patients, the less time I have to spend with those who
truly need to see a doctor.

Before we can determine a treatment in modern medicine, we must first diagnose the underlying illness. Likewise, when we seek treatment for our souls, we must first understand that we have a spiritual sickness. We need to know that we are sinners in need of a Savior. If we self-righteously think that we have it all together, in effect we're saying that we don't need Jesus. But if we know we're sick and dying, and we want treatment, then we will come to Jesus to be healed.

Jesus didn't come to celebrate the righteous; he came to bring healing and redemption to sinners in need of forgiveness. That includes all of us. We need Jesus to cure our sin problem.

TODAY'S RX

If you recognize your soul's sickness, spend time today in the presence of the Healer.

Jesus, thank you for leaving your perfect place in heaven to dwell among the sinful and the sick. Thank you for bringing healing to this world and for showing me my need for you. Help me to learn from my past mistakes and follow you.

STRENGTH FOR THE FIGHT, PEACE FOR THE FUTURE

The LORD gives his people strength.
The LORD blesses them with peace.

PSALM 29:11

"I just don't have the strength or will to go one more day," Harvey said. "I'm battle worn. My 'get up and go' done 'got up and went.' I just want to step away from the front lines and have permanent R&R."

Harvey's battle vocabulary was familiar. We often heard similar descriptions from the patients who were referred to our nursing home by the Veteran's Administration. These brave souls had seen the worst of the worst and lived to tell about it. They had post-traumatic stress disorder long before it was even recognized as a syndrome.

Many of the older vets fought in wars that today's teens don't even remember. They fought battles that literally were won in the trenches. In those days, they didn't call it PTSD; they called it shell shock, or combat fatigue, but it's the same thing.

PTSD is an emotional disorder that takes away a soldier's peace and emotional resolve. Recovery takes time and therapy and requires a team of providers coordinating all areas of the veteran's health care. But sometimes even the best medical science and practice can't put all the mental and emotional jigsaw pieces back together again. Only Jesus can.

Most of us have not been in combat, but we've figuratively dodged a few stray bullets in life. Maybe your battle is your marriage, cancer, a friendship, a job, or financial concerns. The effects of the stress can be the same. The constant barrage of stress, fear, and uncertainty wears us out physically, emotionally, and spiritually.

Remember, we were created to live in a garden; yet here we are smack-dab in the middle of the most epic battle ever fought—the battle between good and evil. We continually hear the sirens of jealousy, anger, crime, and disease warning us to take shelter. While the battle with the enemy of our souls rages on, we place our confidence in our holy Commander-in-Chief, who gives us strength when we need it most. We rest in the knowledge that he has already defeated the enemy. The victory is his, and it's also ours for eternity.

TODAY'S RX

Rest in and renew your strength in God's faithful promises. He has defeated the enemy, and the victory is ours.

God, the battles I face on a daily basis are wearing me down. I'm wounded and under attack. Please remind me of the hope I have in you—and your victory over death—to help me through.

DROWNING IN TEARS AND COMPASSION

My life is an example to many, because you
have been my strength and protection.
That is why I can never stop praising you;
I declare your glory all day long.

PSALM 71:7-8

Kurtis and I had been in the same practice years ago. Recently, he and his wife came over for dinner, and we shared memories of the days we'd worked together in the ER.

"You taught me a lot of things when I was working with you," Kurtis said. "But do you know what the most important thing was that you taught me?"

As I tried to think back through twenty years of cases, Kurtis said, "I'll give you a hint. It happened the day that baby drowned."

There had been several children who had drowned over the years I'd practiced medicine in that rural ER, but I distinctly remembered the one he was referring to. A baby, in full cardiac arrest, had been brought in after being rescued from a pond. But despite our best efforts, the Lord had taken this precious baby back into his bosom that day.

"I'm stumped," I said. "Everything we tried that day was pretty much standard procedure. I can't think of anything new or unusual."

"It's what happened after the baby died that stuck

with me," Kurtis said. "What you showed me had nothing to do with medicine and everything to do with practicing medicine."

"What do you mean?"

"You sat down with those young parents, held their hands, and looked them right in their tear-filled eyes. Then you explained that God had their baby. I remember the wife sobbing on your shoulder, and the father crying into his hands. You reached out to touch him and gave him physical comfort. When their crying slowed, you reminded them that this wasn't anyone's fault. Then you asked them to pray with you. I'll always remember the part of your prayer where you said that each day from that day forward would bring all of us closer to the day of reunion with our loved ones who had gone on before us."

I had no idea that I'd made such an impression on Kurtis. I could only give God the glory for being present at that moment and prompting my actions. As today's verse says, he is our strength and protection.

TODAY'S RX

Live out your faith even in the most difficult situations; you never know who might be watching you.

Father, may my faith radiate through my words and actions. May I be a source of comfort to those in need, embracing them in your truth and enfolding them in your love.

SOUL PROVIDER

At that time you won't need to ask me
for anything. I tell you the truth, you will ask
the Father directly, and he will grant your
request because you use my name.

JOHN 16:23

"Sorry to bother you again," Victor said. "But since you're the guy who holds the keys to helping me get well, I need another referral—this time to see a specialist for my back pain."

Victor had struggled with back trouble for several weeks. It had started with mild pain but grew worse until it radiated down his right leg. He was unable to work his factory job, and I had to write an explanatory note so he would be excused without being fired. Next, I wrote a referral for an MRI. Now he was back in my office a third time for authorization to see a neurosurgeon.

Have you ever found yourself in a similar dilemma, having to ask your doctor or insurance provider for permission to treat your basic health-care needs? It's not easy for patients to do this—or for doctors to stay on top of all of the requests.

With all the changes in health care, "Mother, may I" situations are becoming more common. One doctor must determine whether the patient is sick enough to consult with a specialist, who then decides if more diagnostic tests are needed. But to schedule the tests, the patient must get permission from the first doctor. This creates obstacles that can delay the desired outcome of restored good health.

It's easy to see how ridiculous this is in medicine. But how often do we do something similar in our spiritual lives? For example, have you ever asked a friend for advice rather than asking God?

Historically, many people have gone to a priest or pastor for guidance or to request permission to ask God for grace and forgiveness—rather than going to God directly. But Jesus, the Great Physician, is our mediator in heaven. We can go directly to him. He holds the keys to our spiritual health and growth. There is no need for a referral. All our healing comes from his hands.

God's diagnostic and treatment plans have already been written and completed, before we even ask. God is our soul provider.

TODAY'S RX

The Father holds the keys to your healing. Seek him first.

Father, I confess that I often seek advice and counsel from family and friends before coming to you with what's on my mind. Help me to turn to you first when I have important decisions to make, knowing that you've prepared the way for me to go.

SOCIAL SERVICES

God will generously provide all you need. Then you
will always have everything you need and plenty
left over to share with others.

2 CORINTHIANS 9:8

When I was growing up in Plantersville, Alabama, our doors were never locked. In fact, the only door that was ever closed was the screen door, and that was only to keep out the flies.

Screen doors really aren't doors at all. They are invitations to come inside, especially if the smell of freshly baked bread or apple pie is wafting from within. In Plantersville, everyone shared what they had with anyone who was in need or who came by. There always seemed to be plenty, and no one was left out.

This was back before government programs were enlisted to take care of the poor and needy. We were taught to help others because that's just what folks did back then. We helped others and knew they would help us. When a family suffered a tragedy, neighbors near and far fixed meals to feed the family for weeks, months, or however long it took them to get back on their feet.

If a house burned down or a barn was demolished in a storm, the men in town gathered with whatever materials and supplies they had to help rebuild. This was simply our way of life.

But times have changed. Social programs have replaced social neighbors. Doors are no longer open; they are closed and locked to protect the material goods that people have amassed. And even that isn't enough to protect our stuff. Now, we install alarms and cameras to keep thieves and the needy away. Our world seems less interested in sharing our stuff and more interested in sharing our opinions on social media.

We used to depend on God to supply all our needs. Today's verse says that he will provide so generously that we will always have more than enough to share with others. But, somehow, we've left that promise behind a locked door. Perhaps we've left God behind too.

We need to remember that God doesn't want—or need—to be locked up and protected. He beckons us from the screen door with a pie in the oven. His invitation is always open for all who care to enter.

TODAY'S RX

Open hands lead to open hearts. The more we share, the better our world will be.

God, help me to have more of a servant's heart and provide for those in need. You are glorified in these kind acts, and I desire to reflect your loving nature.

SING TO THE LORD
YOUR SONG

There I will go to the altar of God, to God—
the source of all my joy. I will praise you
with my harp, O God, my God!

PSALM 43:4

Since the beginning of time, music has been a part of God's creation. I have heard that in the original Hebrew language of the Bible, it says that God sang us into existence. Can you imagine that? On earth, we occasionally refer to an accomplished singer as someone who has "a heavenly voice." But what must the voice of heaven itself sound like?

If it was through music that we were created, it makes sense that music would also sustain us and heal us. As a doctor, I recognize the importance of music in the healing process. The medical literature is full of studies of how music can help us to heal. Healers who want to specialize in this area can get a degree in music therapy.

We were created in God's image, so it is no surprise that we also create through music. From a mother's simple lullaby as she sings her baby to sleep to a symphony of musicians playing their parts to create something bigger than themselves, music reminds us that we are creators too.

I've been blessed with children, and now children-in-law, who are gifted in the art of music.

It's hard to imagine our lives without music. One of my good friends, professional musician Steven Curtis Chapman, continues to write some of the most uplifting songs this world has ever heard. The highest praise a musician can receive is that his or her song has touched someone else's soul. I imagine that's also why God loves it when we sing to him—because our souls reach out to him.

As a doctor, I know there won't be a need for my services in heaven. So rather than risk unemployment, I am practicing my singing in the hopes that one day I can get a job in the heavenly choir.

TODAY'S RX

Worship the Creator through music. Sing a song today that heals your heart, and it just may heal your body, too.

God, thank you for the gift of music and how it is uplifting to so many. May I always sing songs of praise and worship to you.

GUIDANCE COUNSELOR

The LORD says, "I will guide you along
the best pathway for your life.
I will advise you and watch over you."
PSALM 32:8

"What do you mean I failed the test? I've never failed a test in my life!" I said, protesting much more than the moment called for.

"It was only an eye test," the doctor said. "You'll get past it."

What he didn't know was that failing the eye exam was the only thing preventing me from becoming an Air Force pilot. I was eighteen years old and poor. Becoming a pilot was the only way I knew to get off the farm and fly away from the memories of my past.

I went to see my college professor and told him what had happened. "You could get another job in the military," he suggested.

"If I can't fly, I don't want another job in the military!"

"Then what do you want to do?"

"I don't know."

"You would make a good dentist," he said.

I returned a month later, even more upset than I'd been the first time. "I failed that test, too, because I couldn't see the pictures!"

"Ahh," he said. "You should take the MCAT to get into medical school. It doesn't have all of that visual perception stuff on it. You would make a fine doctor."

So, for the third time in three months, I went to take a test that would determine the direction of my life. I didn't have a lot of hope.

A few weeks later, the results came in the mail. I had passed! Apparently, being able to see well is not a requirement for becoming a doctor.

Looking back, it's easy for me to see how God guided me toward the path he had for my life, even though I had other plans and was an atheist at the time. God nudged me through open doors and nudged me past closed doors and even squeezed me through a window or two. I didn't know he was guiding me, until much later when he and I became reacquainted.

To this day, he continues to guide me through life, and he will until I reach the other side of the veil and see him face-to-face.

TODAY'S RX

If you are surrounded by confusion and closed doors, look to God for guidance.

Give me peace, Lord, when my plans do not always align with yours. Show me the path to take, and restore my hope when doors seem to continually shut in front of me. You know the way, and I will follow after you.

THE WISDOM DIET

Don't be impressed with your own wisdom.
Instead, fear the LORD and turn away from evil.
Then you will have healing for your body
and strength for your bones.

PROVERBS 3:7-8

Betsy had been a patient of mine for years. And for as long as I'd known her, she had struggled with her weight, trying diet after diet. Most of them didn't work at all. But the only thing worse for her than a diet that failed was one that succeeded—because once she hit her goal, she would return to her normal way of living and gain back everything she'd lost, plus more. Still, it didn't surprise me when she showed up in my office excited about yet another diet plan.

"Dr. Anderson, I lost fifteen pounds the first week! And ten pounds this week! That's twenty-five pounds in two weeks!"

I could tell she was excited. But that was a lot of weight to lose so quickly, and I was concerned.

"Tell me about your new diet."

Betsy described the latest fad diet that was currently getting a lot of attention thanks to a few well-known people who claimed to have lost weight from it. "I think you should recommend it to all your patients!" Betsy said.

However, I knew what Betsy didn't, and I had some well-founded reservations. The plan wasn't well balanced, nor was it sustainable over the long term. In fact, I had recently admitted a patient to the hospital who was in renal failure. When we narrowed down what was causing her kidneys to fail, we linked it to the same diet that Betsy was talking about.

Though Betsy was happy with her results so far, I knew that the diet could do a lot of harm if taken to the extreme. I spent the next few minutes debunking the "wisdom" of what appeared to be such a great thing.

Sometimes we're like that with God, aren't we? We forsake his wisdom in favor of what we think will be a faster, better, or less demanding way to get what we want. But God knows what we don't, and he is the source of all wisdom. That includes nutritional wisdom. If my patients would follow God's dietary wisdom, they would be much healthier.

TODAY'S RX

Eat healthier by choosing fruits and vegetables over processed foods. That one change today will improve your health tomorrow.

Help me to choose healthy ways of living, Lord, that will benefit both my body and my spirit for the long run. Steer me in your direction, and keep me grounded in your Word.

STRENGTH FOR YOUR BATTLE

They did not conquer the land with their swords;
it was not their own strong arm that gave them
victory. It was your right hand and strong arm and
the blinding light from your face that helped them,
for you loved them. . . . Only by your power can
we push back our enemies; only in your name can
we trample our foes. I do not trust in my bow;
I do not count on my sword to save me.

PSALM 44:3, 5-6

When Kellee was diagnosed with ovarian cancer, she knew it wasn't a battle she could fight on her own. Though the available treatments for the disease had progressed enough over the past few years to give Kellee hope for recovery, the battle still would not be easy. The survival rate for the kind of cancer she had was fifty-fifty at best.

"I'm tired. I'm not sure I have the strength to push through," Kellee confided to me one day.

"I understand. This treatment isn't easy. But I believe the Lord will be your strength when you can't muster it on your own," I said. I reminded her that God had gotten her through the first phase, and I was confident he would see her through the next one as well. I told her that God would be with her every step of the way.

During Kellee's treatment, her white blood count

dropped dangerously low. So did her red blood count and platelets. She had to be placed into reverse isolation to protect her from the outside world. During this time, she did not rely on weapons of war or medicine to vanquish her cancerous foe. Instead, she found power in the presence of God.

The battle was long and hard, but it paid off. Weeks later, the final round of chemo was finished. With jubilation in her heart and joy in her eyes, she embraced her family. Together they celebrated her recovery and God's victory.

TODAY'S RX

When the battle seems long and hard, fear not. God's strong arm and the blinding light from his face will help you.

God, I long to be strengthened and revitalized—to celebrate recovery from all that I have faced. Give me the endurance I need to make it through and stand victorious in your sight.

CRUSHED WITHOUT A SCRATCH

He will order his angels to protect you wherever
you go. They will hold you up with their hands so
you won't even hurt your foot on a stone.

PSALM 91:11-12

"The only thing I remember," Susan said, "was seeing everything go by in slow motion. I heard the tires screeching, and I smelled smoke. Pretty soon, there was so much smoke that I couldn't breathe. The stench of diesel fuel and burning rubber filled my nostrils."

The pictures of the car that Susan showed me on her phone were astounding. The entire front end of the car was demolished. Very little of the vehicle was even recognizable. The roof was gone, as well as both front tires.

"A semi jackknifed in front of us, and the only place to go was underneath it. I should have been killed or at least mangled as much as the car. I still don't understand why there isn't a scratch on me. I thought that little red car was going to be my coffin."

"Good thing you were the only one in the car," I said.

"But I wasn't. The whole family was headed to a revival when this happened. My husband and two children were also in the car. Satan wanted to destroy what we were doing."

"How in the world did four occupants survive that crash?" I said. The entire car was crushed and compressed—there didn't seem to be any room in there for four people to survive, let alone not be hurt.

"God intervened in a mighty way," Susan said. "He not only spared my life, but my family's lives as well."

I was shocked and amazed. It was nothing short of a miracle that Susan and her family were able to continue their journey after the detour they took under the carriage of that semitrailer. God was definitely with them that day. It was obvious that only he and his angels could have protected them in such a catastrophic situation.

TODAY'S RX

God is sovereign, and he performs miracles of healing and protection.

Lord, I praise you for how you work miracles. Thank you for taking me under your wing and protecting me this day. Please watch over my loved ones and keep them safe as well.

I WILL RETURN

"I will return to you about this time next year,
and your wife, Sarah, will have a son!" Sarah was
listening to this conversation from the tent.

GENESIS 18:10

"Doc, I'm afraid my life hasn't always been on the straight and narrow," Sean said. It was his first visit, and we were going over his past medical history. "When I was younger, I was an IV drug user, and I contracted hepatitis C."

Looking Sean in the eye, I could instantly see his anguish. He had repented of his old ways but was left with the consequences of those former sins. "Hepatitis C is a virus that attacks the liver, and in some cases, it can cause cirrhosis and liver failure," I said.

"Yeah. That's exactly what I'm afraid of. My cousin just died of liver failure. I was there with him, and he suffered tremendously. Can you make sure I don't suffer?"

I thought about how hard it must be to live with such severe consequences. "There are some new treatments in the final stages of testing by the FDA. The results look promising. Let's see if you qualify for one of those studies. But I don't want to get your hopes up."

"I'm willing to try," Sean said. "Even if I'm in the control group and get the placebo, maybe they will learn something that can help someone else."

In today's verse, the verb "I will return" in Hebrew means "to intervene in someone's life to change his or her destiny." Certainly, if Sarah had a baby, it would forever change her life. At the time, though, she had a lot of doubts about whether that would happen.

Often, my patients face the same kinds of doubts about their treatments, and so do I. Until they return to my office, we can't be sure whether the treatment is working. When Sean qualified for the new treatment in a double-blind trial, we didn't know which drug he had received. When I saw him several weeks after he started the trial, he seemed somewhat improved, but we still didn't know for sure.

When Sean returned to my office a year later, it was evident that he had been cured. His destiny had been changed because God had intervened, and his life was starting anew.

TODAY'S RX

Be alert to new ways in which God may want to intervene and change your destiny.

God, I praise you for providing for my needs. When I have doubts, you have answers, and I know my life is in good hands. Thank you for setting my path straight and leading the way.

ONLY GOD'S PROMISES

Reassure me of your promise, made to those
who fear you. . . . Remember your promise
to me; it is my only hope.

PSALM 119:38, 49

Remember the TV quiz show *Who Wants to Be a Millionaire?* The game offered contestants three lifelines if they didn't know the answer to a question. The first lifeline was to phone a friend, the second was to poll the audience, and the third option was to have the producers narrow the possible answers down to two, creating a fifty-fifty chance. If I were playing, I'd want God to be my "phone a friend" lifeline! I would gladly give up the other two options if I could phone God anytime I had a question.

I know that's how Allen must have felt. When I walked into his hospital room, he turned and said, "Dr. Anderson, the oncologist told me that I have a fifty-fifty chance of survival if I do chemo. But here's the thing. I had a friend who had the same kind of cancer, and he did the chemo and then got very sick and died anyway. I'm not sure I want to go through what he did. Do you think I could get a second or third opinion and go with the majority vote?"

The oncologist had given him a fifty-fifty chance, and now Allen wanted to poll an audience of other oncologists to see what the majority would say. I guess that made me the "phone a friend" option.

Allen was using all of his lifelines, but his concern was more important than any game show question. The answer he chose could determine the outcome of his life.

"Allen, I think you're smart to ask all these questions and get as much information as you can. We can get a second opinion and a third if that's helpful. The Bible says that with many counselors there is much wisdom. But let me just say that we don't know anything for certain. Even something that sounds as mathematical as a fifty-fifty chance is only a guess. The numbers come from large population studies, and even there we see notable variations. I recommend that we look at the odds optimistically and pray that God will intervene and heal you 100 percent, not 50 percent."

Though medical science can make mathematical predictions, our hope isn't in science; it's in the God of hope.

TODAY'S RX

God alone knows best, and his promises bring hope.

God, what a comfort it is knowing I'm saved by your grace. Because of your Son, my debt is paid in full—not half or any other amount. You have preserved my life and given me hope.

Day 75

INCREDIBLE SACRIFICES

God also bound himself with an oath, so that
those who received the promise could be perfectly
sure that he would never change his mind. So God
has given both his promise and his oath. These two
things are unchangeable because it is impossible
for God to lie. Therefore, we who have fled to him
for refuge can have great confidence as we hold
to the hope that lies before us.

HEBREWS 6:17-18

"I'm wondering if I can get along with just one
kidney," Steve said.

"Why are you asking?"

"My sister has renal failure, and she has to go on
dialysis until she can get a kidney transplant. I'd like
to give her one of mine. I've prayed about it, and I
think it's the right thing to do."

Steve had obviously thought long and hard
about this decision and had prayed for wisdom, but
I warned him that donating a kidney is a serious and
complex business.

"First we would need to see if you two are a
match. If so, we can explore other questions, such
as whether your current kidney function is healthy
enough. We need to make sure you can live a long
and healthy life with just one kidney."

"Let's do it!" Steve said.

The test results showed that Steve was a perfect
match for his sister. In addition, his kidney function

was healthy; he could make the donation without compromising his own health.

"I know you love your sister very much, and this is an admirable thing you're doing, but you have to remember that this sacrifice of love is forever. There's no turning back once you decide to move forward."

"I've never been more certain about anything," Steve said without hesitation. "I just want my sister to have her old life back."

Giving a kidney to someone in need is a sacrificial act of love, but it pales in comparison to the sacrifice that Jesus made on the cross. He willingly gave up his life, not to preserve our old lives, but so that we could have *new* life in him.

TODAY'S RX

When we lovingly sacrifice for others, we do what Jesus first did for us.

Father, help me to give to others as you have given to me. Help me not to cling to worldly goods, but to share them with others in need. I desire to have a sacrificial spirit like yours.

SET ASIDE YOUR ANSWERS TO HEAR HIS

Harden the hearts of these people. Plug their ears
and shut their eyes. That way, they will not see with
their eyes, nor hear with their ears, nor understand
with their hearts and turn to me for healing.

ISAIAH 6:10

Early one morning, Mike called my office. He was
having stomach pains and was convinced he had a
rare form of cancer. He insisted on seeing me that day.

When he arrived that afternoon, he had a stack of
printouts listing diseases and symptoms that matched
his experience. He told me about the research he'd
done online and the diagnoses he'd considered. He
firmly believed that he had a particularly nasty—and
rare—cancer, and he was understandably stressed.

When I asked about his symptoms, Mike listed
several things that had been bothering him. Though
some of his symptoms were consistent with the
cancer he had discovered on the Internet, I was able
to quickly rule it out. Ultimately, it was something
much easier to diagnose and treat—irritable bowel
syndrome—but it had worsened as a result of his
worrying. After we discussed a treatment plan, Mike
went home with a relieved smile on his face.

Coming up with our own answers to physical or
spiritual problems can often make us anxious. That's
why I love the opening line of Psalm 46:10: "Be still,

and know that I am God!" Even with my years of medical training and experience, I still rely on God to guide me and to give me insight into the diseases or injuries that cause my patients' symptoms.

When we go to God with our own list of answers, telling him what we think is wrong, we miss an opportunity to hear his wise diagnosis. Instead, we should present him with our spiritual symptoms—whether we're experiencing fear, anger, or anxiety—and allow his Word to diagnose our spiritual diseases. No matter if our pain is physical or emotional, God is the one who can heal us. Sometimes he uses doctors—or even an article on the Internet—but if we want to be blessed by his wisdom, we must go to him prepared to listen.

TODAY'S RX

When you hear hoofbeats, you're more likely to see a horse than a zebra, so take a deep breath before diagnosing yourself with something you read about on the Internet.

Thank you, God, that you have the answers to all my needs. Help me to be still before you, listening for your wisdom as I go through times of worry.

HE ALWAYS ANSWERS

I am praying to you because I know you will
answer, O God. Bend down and listen as I pray.

PSALM 17:6

"When you told me I had ALS, you said my prognosis
was about two years. Is that still what you think?"
Albert asked.

"Only God knows the hour, but based on those
who've been in similar circumstances, I think that's
about right."

Albert was a large, burly man who spoke with a
deep-toned voice. Today that voice was filled with
resignation. His petite wife sat quietly at his side,
taking it all in. Of all the diagnoses I give my patients,
ALS, or Lou Gehrig's disease, is one of the worst. I
knew how many challenges the couple would face in
the next few months.

"Now Albert, that's just what the textbooks say.
But God is still God, and it doesn't mean we can't
pray for a miracle."

"My wife and I pray every day that when I wake
up in the morning, I won't have this cross to bear.
But so far, God has answered differently."

Albert was right. It wasn't that God didn't answer
their prayers; it was just that he hadn't answered them
the way they had hoped.

I've begun to understand that, even when God's
answers are not what we hoped for, there *is* a reward

that comes later. Jesus himself experienced this right before he went to the cross. He asked his Father in heaven to remove the cup of suffering from him if it was aligned with his will. The answer Jesus got was not the one he hoped for. But he followed his Father's plan anyway. He knew the reward that would come at the end of his mission.

When you ask God for something, do you get disappointed or even angry when the outcome is not what you wanted or expected? Do you sometimes misinterpret God's answer as not answering?

Albert's journey was hard, but he understood that God always answered his prayers, even when the answers weren't what he had hoped for. And this knowledge transformed his prayers. Over time, his prayers were transformed as he learned to pray for God's will first and foremost.

Albert was eventually healed of ALS but not here on earth. The reward for his faithfulness came when he entered eternity.

TODAY'S RX

God always hears and answers our prayers. And God always keeps his promises.

God, thank you for bending down and listening to my prayers. You hear my praises and my cries, and you answer faithfully all I ask. Help me to be patient and steadfast in my faith as I wait on you.

REMEMBER ME AND SHOW ME FAVOR

Remember me, Lord, when you show favor to
your people; come near and rescue me. Let me
share in the prosperity of your chosen ones. Let me
rejoice in the joy of your people; let me praise you
with those who are your heritage.

PSALM 106:4-5

A big-city hospital can be a scary place for some of
my patients, and sometimes it can be overwhelming
for me, too.

One day, I called the regional hospital on
behalf of Diana, who had presented in our ER with
heart attack symptoms and needed to be seen by a
cardiologist. The staff said they were full, but they
would do what they could.

By the time I reached the hospital, Diana had
been moved to the last room at the end of a very
long hallway, in a far corner of the hospital. It was a
miserable experience walking through endless cold
and sterile hallways looking for her room.

When I arrived, it felt isolated and dark with only
a single small window, but I knew it was the only
available room.

"I'm so glad to see you!" Diana said. "You're the
first familiar face I've seen here!"

I knew what she meant; she was the first familiar
face I'd seen, as well.

Diana looked frightened as I sat down beside her bed. "Don't worry. I know this place is big and can seem scary. But God is with you, and he allowed me to be here to help you navigate through the confusing maze of hallways and all the paperwork."

She smiled.

"The specialists here are top-notch," I said. "And the cardiologist will be here in a short while." As a country doctor, my presence at the bigger hospital was often more about making the patients comfortable than for medical purposes.

Diana and I chatted until the cardiologist arrived. He ordered some tests, and we learned that Diana had a cardiac arrhythmia. In the cardiology lab, they were able to quickly diagnose and fix the abnormality in her heart's electrical system.

In medicine, we all do what we can to make our patients feel better. The cardiologist was there to steady her heartbeat, and I was there to steady her nerves.

TODAY'S RX

Don't be afraid. Wherever you are, the Lord is with you, and you are not alone. He will never leave you.

Lord, help me to be still and trust in you when the path ahead is frightening. I know you're beside me, lighting the way.

THE BRAVE BOY BORN TO HELP OTHERS

Wait patiently for the LORD. Be brave and
courageous. Yes, wait patiently for the LORD.

PSALM 27:14

Karen was twenty weeks pregnant when we found
out that our unborn son, David, would be born with
a bilateral cleft lip and palate. The face ultrasound
was new—only having been used for a few months
at the time—otherwise we wouldn't have known that
early.

We didn't have a lot of information, so our minds
were filled with questions. What caused this? What
else might be wrong with him? When can we fix it?
Who will fix it? Where will the surgery have to be
done? We prayed each day that God would direct
our paths and bring the puzzle pieces together in due
time.

When David was born, we were blessed with
a screaming, bouncing baby boy who was healthy
except for the cleft lip and palate.

Karen had done part of her master's work in
nutrition on special feeding problems in newborns,
so she was prepared. I had done extra rotations in
plastic surgery as a family practice resident, so I knew
who to call. God had prepared us years before by
answering many of our questions before we even
asked.

The corrective treatments required patience. The plastic surgeon told us to be prepared for eighteen years' worth of treatments and surgery for David. His cleft lip and palate had a tremendous impact on him but not in the way we were expecting.

Last year, David graduated from Samford University with a degree in nursing. He's hoping to go back for more study so he can become a nurse anesthetist. He told us, "After thirty-five surgical procedures, the person who always gave me the most hope and comfort was the anesthetist who put me to sleep and woke me up. I want to be that person for other people, to help them be brave and courageous when they are facing those same fears."

TODAY'S RX

Bravery develops with time and experience of God's faithfulness.

Help me to see the bigger picture behind my illness, God. Use this often-painful experience to shape my life going forward, so I may see the good that will come from it and glorify you.

THE MIRACULOUS TURNAROUND

Through Christ you have come to trust in God.
And you have placed your faith and hope in
God because he raised Christ from the dead
and gave him great glory.

1 PETER 1:21

"Ma'am, your son is very, very sick. Do you know what happened?"

"I don't know," Barb said through her tears. "He's been struggling to fit in at school this year. We just moved, hoping that would help. His old friends just hung out together and got high. I always told him that nothing good would come from that."

She started to cry harder.

"Colin came home last night from his AA meeting, and he seemed on top of the world. He played with his little sister, and we told him how proud we were of him. He was doing better and getting his life back on track. Around nine, he went upstairs to his room. I knew he was tired, and I didn't think anything about it until this morning when my husband tried to wake him up. Then he started CPR while I called 911 . . . is he going to be okay?"

"It's too early to tell," I said. "His oxygen saturation levels were dangerously low. We've got him intubated, and there's a machine helping him breathe, so right now his blood pressure and his pulse are good. We need to transfer him to downtown Nashville to the ICU—"

"I just want him to be okay," Barb sobbed as she watched the EMTs wheel Colin out to the ambulance.

"Could we stop right now and pray for your son and your family?" I asked.

Barb nodded.

After I prayed, asking God to surround and protect Colin, Barb and her husband left to follow the ambulance. But things didn't look good for Colin.

The next day, I dreaded getting the report from the ICU. But when the call came, the pulmonologist sounded giddy. "There was a miracle in bed 15!"

"Colin, the young man with the overdose?"

"Yes! He woke up this morning and smiled at me."

"What?"

"We took him off life support, and he's doing great. He should be out of the hospital and back home by the end of the week."

Without a doubt, I knew that Colin's life had been snatched out of the jaws of death and that God alone deserved the glory.

TODAY'S RX

God has the power, and the will, to snatch us from the very jaws of death.

God, you are mighty to save. Thank you for the miracles you perform. Even when I am disobedient, you show your grace and favor to me. I am forever grateful.

HEALING POWER OF TEARS

You keep track of all my sorrows. You have
collected all my tears in your bottle. You have
recorded each one in your book.

PSALM 56:8

As a young man growing up on a farm, I had no
idea what the phrase "I just need a good cry to feel
better" meant. It wasn't until I got married and had
three daughters that I understood the importance of
that statement.

Men are sometimes reluctant to show their
emotions. We think of shedding tears as being weak.
We'll often just buck up and swallow our emotions,
internalizing the things that need to be brought up
and dealt with.

Generally, women are much better communicators
—especially when it comes to feelings. They're much
less reserved about pouring out their hearts and
souls. Over the years of being in a predominantly
female house, I have seen, up close and personal, the
positive effects of crying at the right time for the
right reasons.

God created us to have emotions, and tears can
be very therapeutic. In fact, even Jesus wept at the
death of Lazarus.

In addition to the spiritual benefits, tears have
documented healing properties. For example,

our tears are similar in composition to the saline solution we use to resuscitate people when they are about to code. And biologically, the release of tears is accompanied by chemical changes in the brain.

There are times when we need to cry and times when we need to cry out to God and ask him to intercede for our needs. Healing tears can be used to reset our emotional center toward all that is good and godly.

And perhaps you'll learn what I learned: Understanding our own tears can help us to understand the tears of others.

TODAY'S RX

Know that it is healing to release your fears with tears.

Thank you, Father, for hearing my cry when I am feeling sad. I take comfort in knowing that you're alongside me during my time of need and that none of my sorrow is ever in vain.

Day 82

MIDNIGHT
IN THE ER

Weeping may last through the night, but joy
comes with the morning. . . . You have turned my
mourning into joyful dancing. You have taken away
my clothes of mourning and clothed me with joy,
that I might sing praises to you and not be silent.
O LORD my God, I will give you thanks forever!

PSALM 30:5, 11-12

Graveyard shifts in the emergency room can bring
out the worst cases. It seems that patients with
strokes and heart attacks arrive at the same time as
victims of horrific car accidents. Crying babies can
be heard above all the usual noises, and the line for
X-rays can get lengthy with all the broken bones.
During the overnight shift, weariness sets in for both
the sick and those who treat them.

"Will this pain ever end?"

"Will this night ever be over?"

"How long will our weeping last?"

Waiting for answers while the night grows longer
can cause both patients and providers to lose patience.
But as a doctor, I know that when dawn bursts over
the eastern sky, our cortisol levels start to rise as well.
We experience a kind of rush of adrenaline. With
this boost of God-given energy from the body, we
can often experience a lift in our moods. We begin
the new day with hope.

During those rosy-pink hours of early daylight, doctors often find that they are able to wean patients off of artificial systems and oxygen tubes that have kept them alive. They have made it through their dark night, and during the first hours of light, they begin their journey back to independence.

TODAY'S RX

No matter how dark the night or how loud the cries, morning releases mourning and restores the soul to new life.

God, thank you for piercing the darkness with your light. You reenergize me daily with your hope. This world does its best to cloud my vision, but you lift the fog and show me your great love.

HIDDEN DEVILS

Jesus went around doing good and healing all who
were oppressed by the devil, for God was with him.

ACTS 10:38

As a third-year resident in family medicine, I had
the opportunity to serve as the medical director of
a mental health hospital in Jackson, Tennessee. The
duties, for the most part, were routine. It was my job
to make sure that the patients were medically healthy.
If we had to admit someone, it was typically because
his or her outpatient treatment plan had failed.

Larry was an exception. He was sent to the
hospital by a court order because he thought he was
possessed by Satan. An unusually large man with a
massive forehead, Larry had had periodic outbursts
toward his family, and the police had been called to
his house on several occasions for domestic violence.

As I examined him, he seemed to look right
through me—peering off into a world that the rest
of us couldn't see. He had been diagnosed with
schizophrenia, but his medical history was unusual.
His symptoms had appeared much later in life than
was typical for schizophrenia. Larry also suffered
from migraines, and there was something unusual
about the size of his hands and feet.

When his lab work came back, I could see that
he had diabetes mellitus and renal failure. There
were now more questions in his chart than answers.

I spoke with the psychiatrist who was treating Larry's mental illness and requested a CT scan of Larry's head. When the results came back, we were able to see for the first time what was going on. It turned out that Larry had a pituitary tumor that was causing acromegaly—a hormonal disease that causes growth hormones to be released long after the body should have stopped growing. This explained the unusual size of his face, feet, and hands. They had continued to grow well into adulthood.

We began treatment on the tumor immediately, and within three weeks, his "schizophrenia" symptoms improved. God had removed "the devil" that had tormented this man for so many years.

TODAY'S RX

Regardless of your affliction, whether spiritual or physical, God wants to heal you. Sometimes he uses a pastor, and other times he uses a physician.

God, only you can see my innermost parts. Please detect in me where I need healing, both in body and spirit. I give myself to you.

Day 84

COME DIRTY
AND GET CLEAN

I will save them from their sinful apostasy.
I will cleanse them. Then they will truly be
my people, and I will be their God.

EZEKIEL 37:23

Nick had once owned his own business and had been a well-respected member of the community. But as I watched the prison guard escort him down the hall, what defined his life now was an orange jumpsuit. Once Nick was settled in the exam room, the guard walked out and closed the door.

"I can't take it!" Nick said. "This is my third DUI, and they sentenced me to eleven months and twenty-nine days. That's a year in jail, and it will ruin me! What am I going to do? I've already lost my business, and now my wife is leaving with the kids."

"I can help you medically, Nick, but only God can restore what's broken in you. I know he can restore your health and life while you're in jail. If you let him, he can work a miracle."

Nick settled back in his chair and seemed to think about what I had said.

"St. Paul spent time in prison," I said. "In fact, God spoke to him there, many, many times. I'm going to pray that God speaks to you, as well."

What in your life is keeping you in prison? What idols distract you from the love of God? Whether it's a relationship, an illness, an addiction, or a preoccupation with the wrong things, God wants to cleanse your lost and broken soul and restore you to wholeness.

A year later, Nick came to see me in my office—not as a new patient, but as a new man. He had a spring in his step and a lift in his voice as he told me how God had not only forgiven him, but had also restored him to his family.

"I began reading the Bible again," he said. "And you were right. That jail time saved my life."

I asked Nick about his plans for the future.

"I'm already working," he said with a grin. "I'm a drug and alcohol counselor at a rehab facility. I get paid to bring the hope of new life through Jesus Christ to those who need a fresh start."

TODAY'S RX

It's easy to become a prisoner to the idols in our lives. Ask God to cleanse you and restore your love for him.

God, I pray that you would remove any unhealthy habits that have become a stronghold on my life. Take away the distractions and idols that keep me from finding my identity in you. I desire to start fresh and be made whole.

WISE ADVICE FOR
A HEALTHY LIFE

Those who trust their own insight are foolish,
but anyone who walks in wisdom is safe.

PROVERBS 28:26

"My wife made me come in. She's the one who thinks I need a checkup. I haven't been to a doctor in more than twenty years, and I'm doing just fine. Nothing hurts, and I pretty much do whatever I want."

Elmer's body told a different story from the one he was voicing to me. He was fifty-three but looked sixty-five. He was fifty pounds overweight, and his blood pressure was elevated.

"Let's get a medical history on you and run some tests, and then we'll see," I said. "Does anyone in your family have a history of diabetes, heart disease, or cancer?"

"Yeah, Daddy died of a heart attack when he was fifty-two, and my brother died last year of a heart attack. I think he was fifty-three. My momma had diabetes, but that was only 'cause she was fat like me."

I could tell I had my work cut out for me. Elmer seemed blissfully unaware of the connection between the premature deaths of his close family members and his own prospects for long-term survival. And he was oblivious to his own body's warning signs.

His tests for diabetes and cholesterol both came back abnormally high.

"Elmer, you're not doing as well as you think you are," I said, showing him the results. "You're behind in your health care, and if you don't change, you'll likely die before you're fifty-five. You have a lot of work to do. The good news is that, if you listen to me and work hard, you can fix a lot of this."

"You've got my full attention, Doc. I've got kids that I want to see get married, and I want to be a grandfather one day."

I prescribed medication for his blood pressure, his diabetes, and his cholesterol. We talked about how he needed to quit smoking and stop eating so much processed food. Elmer was obviously surprised by everything I said.

"Am I doing anything right?" he asked.

"Yes. You listened to your wife when she sent you in for a checkup. Be sure to thank her when you get home."

TODAY'S RX

Seek wise counsel and follow the advice you're given if you want to live a healthier life.

Help me to be obedient in all aspects of my life, Lord, by listening to my doctor's advice, along with what your Word tells me. I desire to be healthy in body, mind, and spirit.

Day 86

THE BLESSINGS OF CONTENTMENT

*From his abundance we have all received one
gracious blessing after another.*

JOHN 1:16

Bernie, my first patient of the morning, took one look at me and said, "You look tired."

He was right. I knew I did. It was a Monday morning, and I had just finished a weekend shift in the ER.

"For an old watermelon farmer, I'm doing fine," I said.

Bernie laughed.

Every day I feel blessed beyond measure. Growing up, I had much less materially than I do now. But even back then, I remembered being content and happy with what God had given me.

Though my fatigue was showing that morning, it didn't keep me from counting all the ways God has blessed this poor country boy from Alabama. For example, I love serving underprivileged country folks just like the ones I grew up with. God has given me an amazing wife and four wonderful children, and we all have more than enough clothes and food and a comfortable home. The kids are all healthy and doing well, and we have friends at both church and school.

"Enough about me, how are you and your kids doing?" I asked Bernie.

I listened as Bernie told me about his family. We were both blessed not only to have our families and our jobs, but also to have grown up in America, where we can take advantage of the opportunities that this country offers. No matter what troubles we face, our blessings certainly outweigh them.

Our contentment shouldn't be determined by the idols we have created. It should come from our appreciation of what God has done for us. Even on a Monday morning when I am tired from working all weekend, I can still say that God has blessed me, and I am content.

TODAY'S RX

If you search for contentment, you may never find it. But if you count your blessings, you surely will.

Father, help me to remember and be thankful for all the blessings you have bestowed on me. Even in the difficult times, may I never forget all you have done for me.

Day 87
LAST HOPE

Jesus said, "Someone deliberately touched me,
for I felt healing power go out from me."
LUKE 8:46

Elaine sat quietly in the corner of the waiting room. When her name was called, she got up slowly from her chair and made her way down the hall to the exam room.

"I don't know what to do," she said. "I'm swelling all over. It's worse in my legs, and I'm losing my strength. I'm always short of breath, and I don't think I can take another step."

We helped her into the room, and I began my exam.

"I've seen at least ten doctors before I came to see you, and they all just shook their heads. They couldn't give me an answer. You're my last hope."

She had visited a number of specialists, and most of the doctors on her list were much more qualified than I was. If they hadn't turned up anything specific, how could she expect me to have an answer? I was just a country doctor.

But I was also a believer. "Let's pray that God will show us what's wrong," I suggested. "Perhaps he can use one of the tests I'll run to give us some answers."

After we prayed together, I said, "I'll track down the test results from the other doctors you've visited, and I'll order some additional ones. Once we have all the results, we'll see what God can tell us."

During the week, while I pondered Elaine's condition, I thought about the bleeding woman who had reached out to touch the robe of Jesus. I'm sure she had sought help from other healers and that none had been able to help her. As she approached Jesus, he was her last hope.

A week later, with the test results in hand, I had an idea of what was causing Elaine's symptoms. She had nephritic syndrome, which her nephrologist later determined was due to abnormal protein flowing through her blood. After another week, we were able to confirm a diagnosis of amyloidosis—a condition that causes protein to build up in other tissues and organs. Once we identified the cause, we were able to determine the treatment. Elaine needed a bone marrow transplant.

A few months later, Elaine walked into my office and smiled. She was back to her normal self.

TODAY'S RX

When seeking treatment, be persistent, and never give up. Lean on the Lord in faith, and trust his wisdom.

Lord, give me the patience to endure what I'm facing and the reassurance that you have all the answers. I trust in you to direct my path to healing.

RULES ON THE ROAD TO HEALTH

God detests the prayers of a person
who ignores the law.
PROVERBS 28:9

I entered the exam room and shook Kevin's hand. "It's good to see you," I said. "It's been a while since you've been in."

"Yeah, I know. I should have come back like you told me. But, you know, life happens, and I was busy."

"Looking at your chart, I see you've been out of medication. You haven't refilled your prescription in months."

"Yeah, I know. When my prescription ran out, I just stopped refilling it."

"Well, what brings you in today?" I asked.

"I'm having a hard time breathing. It seems like I'm always short of breath, even when I'm not exerting myself."

Kevin's complaints were common. Like most people with medical problems, staying healthy required work. In Kevin's case, he had diabetes, hyperlipidemia, and hypertension. To manage his diseases, he needed to do regular blood sugar and blood pressure checks. He needed to take his medications, follow a prescribed diet, and exercise regularly. But following all of those "rules" wasn't enough. He also had to have regular lab work and visits with his doctor to make sure the prescribed treatment was keeping him on the path to physical health. If not, the health rules he lived by would need to be changed.

Unfortunately, Kevin hadn't obeyed any of the rules he'd been given. As I examined him that day, I realized he was having a massive heart attack. He received immediate intervention to save his life and from that point forward had to follow the rules he had previously ignored. He knew that if he wanted to stay alive, he would have to respect these rules and follow them closely.

If you are driving down the highway and disregard the rules of the road, sooner or later you'll have a major crash. Kevin nearly died because he hadn't obeyed the medical advice he'd been given. In our spiritual lives, just like in medicine, noncompliance can lead to death. The laws of the road, the laws of medicine, and the laws of the Bible are there for our own good. Following them leads to health.

TODAY'S RX

Pay attention to the laws of life. They can keep you alive spiritually and physically.

Father, help me to be wise and live in compliance with your laws. I want to experience more of your glory.

FEAR NOT!

Jesus responded, "Why are you afraid?
You have so little faith!"

MATTHEW 8:26

Scripture repeatedly reminds us to have faith and not to fear.

As a doctor, a lot of my job involves alleviating fear and encouraging faith. When patients are waiting for test results, I tell them not to worry too early. I tell them to wait until we get the results back and know what we're dealing with. When they fear going to the hospital or having surgery, I remind them to trust in the experienced hands of those who will be taking care of them. And with all my patients, I want them to have faith that God is in control.

I understand why my patients fear the unknown and the undiagnosed. When something is amiss with our health, all sorts of thoughts run rampant through our minds. Sometimes the diagnosis is simple and easily treatable. When that happens, a patient's sigh of relief is audible.

"Wow, thanks, I thought it was something more serious!"

Even when the diagnosis is serious or life-threatening, if we put treatment plans in place, the patient has less to fear. Fear grows exponentially when fueled by the unknown.

Maybe that's why Jesus appears so frustrated

with his disciples in today's verse. He was sitting right in front of them. What did they have to fear? They had the answer to all of life's questions in their very presence, and they could ask him anything they wanted. Yet they still doubted, and they still had fear.

With two thousand years of hindsight, it's easy to blame the disciples for their lack of faith. But aren't we also guilty of the same thing? We have all the answers that the early disciples had—*and* we have even more knowledge because we can see life through the historical lens of Scripture. We know that Jesus overcame death on the cross! Why should we ever doubt or fear? He is the way, the truth, and the life!

TODAY'S RX

Seeing Jesus' power throughout history should make us faithful and fearless.

Jesus, be with me when my fears are overwhelming. Help my soul to be still. Remind me of your power and victory over evil, and comfort me in your embrace.

Day 90

GOD'S SUPPLY IS UNLIMITED

When I think of all this, I fall to my knees and
pray to the Father, the Creator of everything in
heaven and on earth. I pray that from his glorious,
unlimited resources he will empower you with
inner strength through his Spirit.

EPHESIANS 3:14-16

If I could choose only one passage of Scripture to
summarize this book, it would be today's verses.

In this world, there are limits to the medical
resources we can provide. In this world, there is not
enough money to pay for every treatment and test
that patients or their doctors want. Your doctor may
prescribe a certain procedure only to find out it's not
covered, it's classified as elective, or it is considered
medically unnecessary. The medical system today
limits us to providing only those things that the
patient needs, according to the powers that be.

Insurance companies, and sometimes government
programs, help to regulate the flow of resources
between the wants and the needs. This is the give-
and-take reality that confronts so many people who
seek treatment for themselves or their loved ones.

Even if we had unlimited financial resources,
we still live in a finite world. Steve Jobs had nearly
unlimited resources with his material wealth, yet

even he wasn't able to buy more time on earth. We all are finite mortals.

When my patients are encumbered by the complexities of the health-care system, I remind them of today's verses. Ultimately, God is our source for all things. His resources are unlimited, and he alone heals. We doctors are just his tools here on earth to help provide temporary cures.

When we look to the infinite, all-powerful, all-knowing God of the universe, we find an endless well of supply. It is from this well that the living waters spring forth to forever heal us.

TODAY'S RX

It only takes a sip of living water for us to never thirst again.

God, there is no one like you. You are infinite, all-powerful, all-knowing, and you love your people with an everlasting love. Thank you for filling my spirit with your living water, reviving me to new life in you.

Scripture Index

Genesis 18:10	Day 73	Psalm 91:11-12	Day 72
Genesis 18:14	Day 42	Psalm 106:4-5	Day 78
Exodus 14:14	Day 47	Psalm 108:1	Day 57
Exodus 15:26	Day 41	Psalm 119:38, 49	Day 74
Deuteronomy 33:27	Day 37	Psalm 119:76-77	Day 53
Nehemiah 8:10	Day 14	Psalm 145:9	Day 32
Psalm 17:6	Day 77	Psalm 147:3	Day 60
Psalm 27:14	Day 79	Proverbs 3:7-8	Day 70
Psalm 29:11	Day 64	Proverbs 4:20-22	Day 1
Psalm 30:5, 11-12	Day 82	Proverbs 12:18	Day 16
Psalm 31:24	Day 4	Proverbs 17:22	Day 24
Psalm 32:8	Day 69	Proverbs 19:23	Day 13
Psalm 33:4	Day 15	Proverbs 28:9	Day 88
Psalm 33:18-19	Day 49	Proverbs 28:26	Day 85
Psalm 34:18	Day 8	Isaiah 6:10	Day 76
Psalm 38:17, 21-22	Day 18	Jeremiah 29:11	Day 62
Psalm 40:2	Day 59	Lamentations 3:21-22	Day 28
Psalm 41:4	Day 9	Lamentations 3:22-23	Day 2
Psalm 42:5-6	Day 11	Ezekiel 37:23	Day 84
Psalm 43:4	Day 68	Ezekiel 47:12	Day 61
Psalm 44:3, 5-6	Day 71	Joel 3:10	Day 22
Psalm 52:8	Day 34	Micah 7:7-8	Day 40
Psalm 56:8	Day 81	Nahum 1:9	Day 31
Psalm 71:7-8	Day 65	Matthew 7:8	Day 5

Matthew 8:16-17	Day 54	Romans 5:5	Day 21
Matthew 8:26	Day 89	Romans 8:2	Day 43
Matthew 12:24	Day 46	Romans 8:31	Day 56
Matthew 14:31	Day 26	Romans 15:13	Day 39
Mark 1:29-31	Day 7	1 Corinthians 15:58	Day 55
Mark 1:32-34	Day 19	2 Corinthians 1:3-4	Day 12
Mark 5:25-28	Day 30	2 Corinthians 9:8	Day 67
Mark 8:23-25	Day 29	Ephesians 1:19-20	Day 58
Luke 4:38-40	Day 44	Ephesians 3:14-16	Day 90
Luke 5:27-32	Day 63	Ephesians 3:20-21	Day 27
Luke 8:46	Day 87	Philippians 1:9	Day 38
Luke 9:6	Day 52	Philippians 4:4	Day 23
Luke 22:32	Day 10	2 Thessalonians 2:16-17	Day 51
John 1:16	Day 86	1 Timothy 4:10	Day 17
John 9:6-7	Day 48	Hebrews 6:17-18	Day 75
John 15:7	Day 25	Hebrews 10:23	Day 36
John 16:23	Day 66	Hebrews 11:1	Day 45
Acts 2:26-27	Day 20	James 1:17	Day 6
Acts 4:30	Day 50	James 5:14	Day 3
Acts 10:38	Day 83	1 Peter 1:21	Day 80
Romans 4:20-24	Day 35	1 Peter 5:10	Day 33

About the Authors

Reggie Anderson, MD, was raised in the small, rural town of Plantersville, Alabama, and has come to embody the small-town wisdom and homespun morality that he grew up with. He graduated from the University of Alabama with a BS in chemistry and an English minor. While attending the University of Alabama Medical School, he met his wife, Karen. He completed his residency in family practice at the University of Tennessee in Jackson.

Reggie and Karen have raised four children, three daughters who are married and a son who is currently in nursing school. He and Karen reside on a farm in Kingston Springs, Tennessee, often opening their home as a refuge for those needing shelter following a natural disaster or other crisis.

Reggie was awarded the Frist Humanitarian Award by the Centennial Medical Center in Nashville. He was chosen from more than nine hundred doctors to be nominated for the national award.

Reggie is a member of the American Academy of Family Physicians and works at the TriStar

Medical Group, where he continues to serve the poor and underprivileged in satellite offices in Ashland City and Kingston Springs, Tennessee. He also serves as chief of staff at TriStar Ashland City Medical Center, as well as the medical director of three nursing homes. Learn more about Reggie at appointmentswithheaven.com.

Jennifer Schuchmann finds great joy in helping authors with compelling messages tell their stories to new audiences.

Notable books include *Taylor's Gift* by Todd and Tara Storch, the story of a couple who donated their daughter's organs after a skiing accident and later met the recipients; *Spirit Rising* by Jim Cymbala, an in-depth look at the Holy Spirit; and *By Faith, Not by Sight* by blind *American Idol* finalist, Scott MacIntyre. A selection of past books includes *One Call Away*, a memoir of Brenda Warner, and *First Things First*, a *New York Times* bestseller by Kurt and Brenda Warner.

Jennifer is the host of *Right Now with Jennifer Schuchmann*, which airs weekly on the NRB Network, Sky Angel satellite, and DIRECTV. She holds an MBA from Emory University, with an emphasis in marketing and communications, and a bachelor's degree in psychology from the University of Memphis. She's been married to David for more than twenty years, and they have a son, Jordan. Learn more about Jennifer at jenniferschuchmann.com, or follow her on Twitter: @schuchmann.